THE LOW-FODMAP DIET FOR BEGINNERS

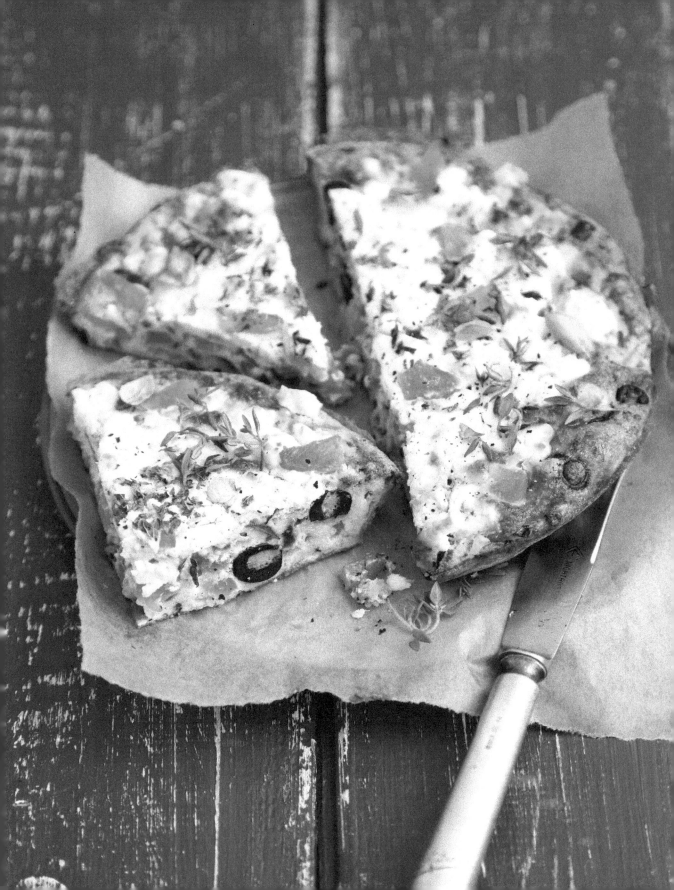

The **Low-FODMAP Diet** *for* **Beginners**

A 7-Day Plan to Beat Bloat and Soothe Your
Gut with Recipes for Fast IBS Relief

MOLLIE TUNITSKY

with Gabriela Gardner, RDN-AP, LD, CNSC

Foreword by Sushovan Guha, MD, PhD

ROCKRIDGE
PRESS

Cover: Banana Pancakes (page 48), Chicken Piccata (page 102); title page: Vegetable Frittata (page 50)

Photo Credits: Photography © Nadine Greeff, cover, pp. vi, ix, 46 & 84, back cover; Foxys Forest Manufacture/Shutterstock.com, cover; Azdora/Shutterstock.com, cover, pp. vii & 2; Rua Castilho/Stockfood, pp. ii & 74; Melina Hammer, pp. vi & 128; Nadine Greeff/Stocksy, pp. vii & 36; Beatrice Peltre/Stockfood, pp. vii & 142; Ruth Black/Stocksy, p. x; Carolin Strothe/Stockfood, p. 14; Gräfe & Unzer Verlag/Janne Peters/Stockfood, p. 28; Eleonora Druzhinina/Shutterstock.com, p. 28; Gareth Morgans/Stockfood, p. 96; Alicia Mañas Aldaya/Stockfood, p. 110.

ISBN: Print 978-1-62315-957-3 | eBook 978-1-62315-958-0

R1

To my loving family and friends for always being there, not just for every stomachache but also for every day.

Thank you to my sweet husband for helping me follow my "gut" and being the ultimate partner in crime.

To anyone who is reading this looking for stomach relief, I know you'll find it, just like I did. Don't give up!

Contents

PART 1
The Low-FODMAP Diet Solution

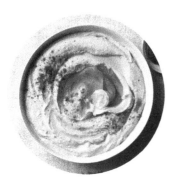
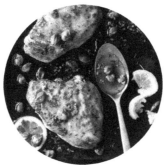
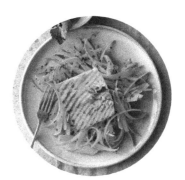

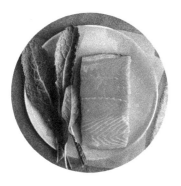
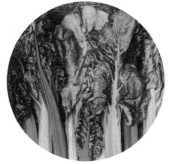
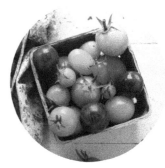

PART 2
Low-FODMAP Recipes

Foreword

Years ago, as a gastroenterology fellow at the University of California, Los Angeles, I was amazed to learn that millions of people in the US suffer from irritable bowel syndrome (IBS). Since completing my fellowship, I've treated many patients with IBS and have seen firsthand the suffering they silently endure. Due to how easily the condition can be exacerbated, IBS is one of the most common conditions that results in visits—often frequent—to clinics and hospital emergency rooms.

I now know that diet plays a major role in instigating or aggravating IBS symptoms, but my medical training did not offer any information on dietary interventions for managing gastrointestinal (GI) disorders, including IBS. I advised my IBS patients to eat less greasy food and more fiber, but I became increasingly frustrated as I saw that this simple advice did not help them in the long run. Finally, the FODMAP-restricted diet, tested in several high-quality clinical trials, came to my attention. Although the results have not been uniformly positive, we know that quality of life measures significantly improve in IBS patients who have followed a FODMAP-restricted diet.

I met Mollie Tunitsky in our GI clinic a few years ago. She had consulted with several local GI specialists about her IBS symptoms and hadn't experienced any substantial improvement. I approached her with a holistic plan to treat IBS with diet, as well as other interventions. She jumped on it and followed the "new" low-FODMAP dietary regimen with the help of Gabriela Gardner, our clinic's registered dietitian nutritionist. Mollie slowly and steadily improved to her "near-normal" status. As Mollie's physician, I am rewarded to know that she is now publishing a book with Gabriela to bring recipes and relief to others.

Although people suffering from IBS are desperate to make a change, they sometimes get the message that a low-FODMAP diet is "too complicated" or "too cumbersome." This book will simply connect with those who are apprehensive about getting started. I read the book intently and believe that it will be a wonderful resource not only for IBS sufferers but also for physicians treating these patients. Although a FODMAP-restricted diet is not a panacea for treating this debilitating

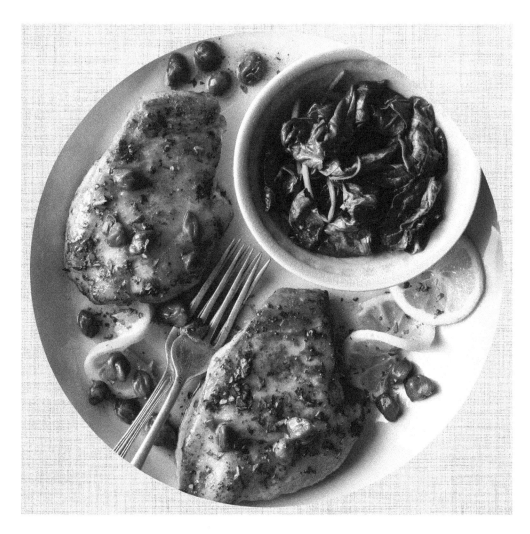

Above: Chicken Piccata, page 102

condition, it certainly helps in several ways, as Mollie notes in the first chapter. I sincerely hope that after reading this book, people who suffer from IBS will incorporate a medically safe, enjoyable, and delicious FODMAP-restricted diet in their daily routine to substantially improve their quality of life.

Have a hearty and healthy meal!

Sushovan Guha, MD, PhD
Associate Professor, Gastroenterology, Hepatology and Nutrition
University of Texas, McGovern Medical School

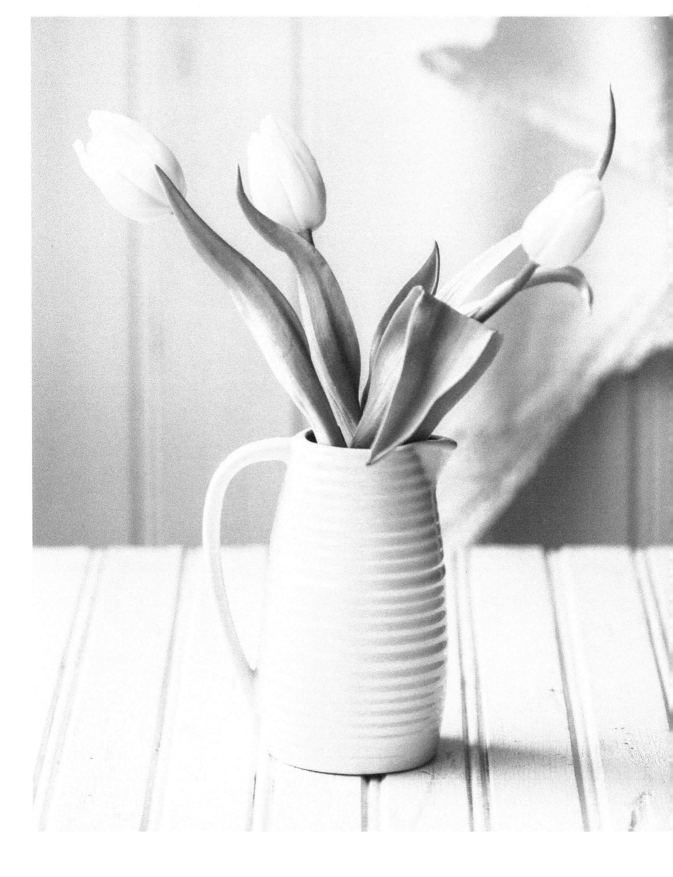

Introduction

$\mathcal{E}$ ver since college, I've had digestive issues, which have ranged on the spectrum from mild to severe. Sometimes they'd be slightly annoying; sometimes I'd have to cancel plans and lie in the fetal position on the living-room couch. There was a lot of anxiety associated with my stomach; I was constantly worried about getting sick while out of the house. I saw a multitude of different gastroenterologists who diagnosed me with irritable bowel syndrome (IBS), but they only asked if I was stressed out, and offered few to no solutions. I even had one doctor tell me to stop eating all fruits and vegetables as one solution. When I asked what I should eat instead, he looked at me like I was the crazy one!

A few years ago, I decided to take my health into my own hands and saw a new gastroenterologist who introduced me to something called the low-FODMAP diet. He also recommended I work with his dietitian. It was the first time in all my years of suffering that someone was interested in what I was eating and how much, instead of just pushing medications at me. I prided myself (I thought) on eating healthy, but it turns out some of those "healthy" foods like apples and cauliflower were high-FODMAP items. After completing the elimination diet, I realized it was those types of foods that were making me feel so sick for all these years.

This is where the low-FODMAP diet and my digestive evolution came into play. It turned my life right-side up in the best way possible, and now I know the same can happen for you. I'm excited for you to dive in and find stomach relief just like I did—probably much more quickly than you ever thought possible!

The goal of this seven-day approach is to avoid all high-FODMAP foods for the entire seven days and see what a difference it makes for your gastrointestinal health. In just one week, you should start to see powerful results and relief. You'll start to understand how your specific issues with IBS, IBD, or general GI sensitivity are triggered—and what you can do to fix them.

PART 1

The Low-FODMAP Diet Solution

This section of the book is for those of you who, like me, are information hounds. I'm always looking for as much information as possible, but I want it to be really clear and really simple. In the next several chapters, I'll explain what FODMAPs are, why they can wreak such havoc on our bodies, and why you won't need to wait weeks or months on a low-FODMAP diet before you start to feel so much better. The truth is, it is a drastic change—at first—so I'll break down the process into a handful of doable steps. I'll introduce you to the meals and snacks (with a shopping list!) that you'll eat over the course of a one-week elimination diet, and then explain how to properly and carefully reintroduce high-FODMAP foods back into your diet.

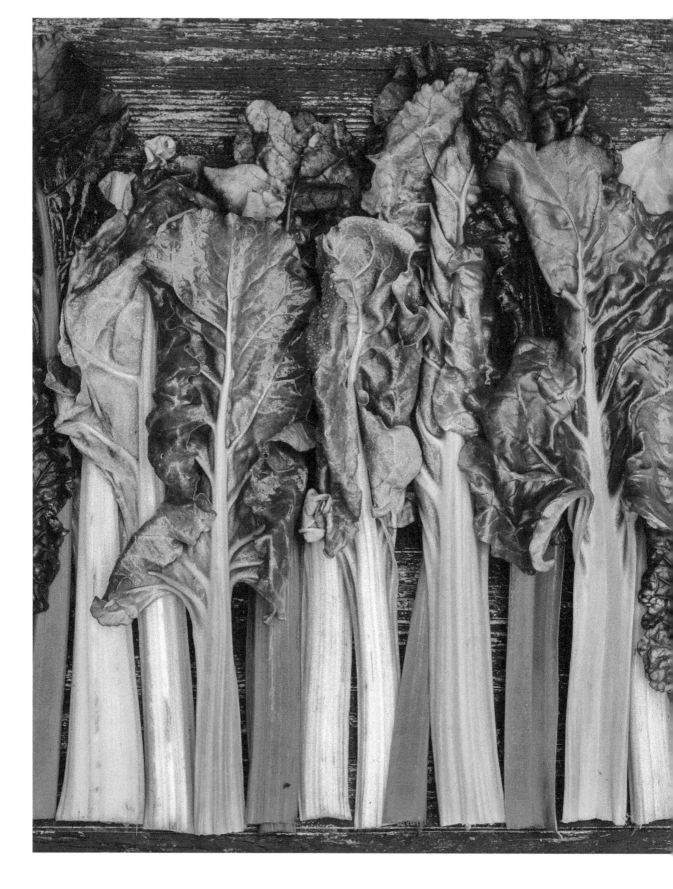

Chapter 1

FODMAPs and You

For so long, I struggled with gastrointestinal issues. As physically uncomfortable as that was, the hardest aspect was feeling isolated, embarrassed, and alone. Have you ever cancelled plans at the last minute because of your stomach troubles? I now know I'm not alone in having done that, and I want to reassure you that you're not either. Whenever I had no choice but to cancel plans last minute, I'd feel guilty, which led to anxiety and stress and—you guessed it—more stomach discomfort. The low-FODMAP diet changed everything for me—not only my GI symptoms but also the associated anxiety and stress. I found relief, and now it's your turn.

Take a moment and reflect on how you feel right now: gassy, bloated, constipated, or just generally uncomfortable? If you're experiencing any of these symptoms, you might find the relief you so desperately want by removing high-FODMAP foods from your diet. You already took the first step by picking up this book. Now think about the possibility of how much better you could feel just seven days from now.

The digestive ailments that used to run my life revolved around gas, bloating, and diarrhea or constipation. Most people I speak with have had these same issues, with some also experiencing constipation. I hear the same statements all the time:

- "I look pregnant after I eat."
- "I have the worst gas, and it's so embarrassing."
- "I'm afraid to go out in case my stomach blows up."

For me, the first step toward healing involved meeting with a gastroenterologist, who ruled out other common digestive disorders. Additionally, I worked with a dietitian, who helped me identify the foods that caused my symptoms. It was a huge shock for me and my family to realize that the food I ate was part of the problem. But I quickly came to learn that it was also part of the solution. I had always been health conscious and watchful of the food I put in my body, but it wasn't until I understood what FODMAPs were and eliminated high-FODMAP foods from my diet that I started feeling better.

What Are FODMAPs?

Simply put, FODMAPs are a type of carbohydrate that some people's bodies don't process very well. You've heard of carbohydrates; they're the molecular compounds that make up foods like bread, rice, potatoes, and sweets, and the human body needs them to store energy and perform other important functions. Sugars and starches are both types of carbohydrates, which are also known as "saccharides," from the Greek word for "sugar." They come in "long chains" (many smaller carbohydrate molecules linked together) and "short chains" (fewer molecules linked together). FODMAPs are short-chain carbohydrates.

FODMAP is an acronym for words I can barely pronounce: **F**ermentable **O**ligo-, **D**i-, **M**ono-saccharides **a**nd **P**olyols. Fortunately, we have the acronym. And here's what it all really means.

FERMENTABLE: Fermentation is the process by which the bacteria that live in the intestines break down carbohydrates. This is a normal part of the digestive process and helps your body get more nutrients and energy out of your food, but it also produces carbon dioxide (gas), hydrogen (gas), and/or methane (gas) in the colon. You read that right: gas, gas, and more gas. If that fermentation happens too fast and/or your body can't absorb the by-products properly, you'll experience symptoms like bloating, abdominal pain, constipation, and diarrhea.

OLIGOSACCHARIDES: Take my word for it—they may be short-chain carbohydrates, but this is not a friendship chain you want to be a part of. This group contains three or more types of sugar linked together—hence the name, which comes from the Greek for "a few sugars." The human body doesn't produce enzymes that can fully break down oligosaccharides, which means there's plenty of it for the bacteria in the intestines to ferment, and too much causes gas, pain, and other symptoms.

- *Fructans* and *galactans* are two categories of oligosaccharides that can be particularly problematic. Foods high in fructans include wheat, rye, onions, and garlic. Foods high in galactans include pulses like lentils, beans, chickpeas, and soybeans.

DISACCHARIDES: The "di" in "disaccharides" indicates that these are two types of sugars (saccharides) linked together. Lactose (which is made of the two monosaccharides galactose and glucose) is the disaccharide you should be most aware of. An enzyme called "lactase" is required to break down this chain. Some people do not produce lactase at all, but its production can also decrease with age or certain digestive disorders.

- *Lactose* is naturally found in milk from cows, goats, and sheep. It is also in milk products like soft cheeses, yogurt, and ice cream.

Note: Sucrose (made of glucose and fructose) is another type of disaccharide. If your body is not able to produce enough sucrase, the enzyme that breaks sucrose down, the result can be gas and bloating. Sucrose is not restricted in the FODMAP diet. If you don't find relief with the FODMAP diet plan, consider discussing with your health-care provider the possibility of a sucrase deficiency.

MONOSACCHARIDES: The "mono" in "monosaccharides" indicates that there is only one type of sugar (saccharide) in this chain of carbohydrates, such as fructose or glucose. If you eat an excess amount of fructose compared to glucose, you might experience fructose malabsorption. This means that the excess fructose moves quickly through the digestive tract without being absorbed as it should, leaving plenty for your gut bacteria to ferment, which causes those painful and embarrassing symptoms.

- *Fructose* in high amounts is found in foods such as honey, mango, and high-fructose corn syrup.

AND . . .

POLYOLS: Due to their chemical makeup, polyols, also known as "sugar alcohols," can't be absorbed by the small intestine. When ingested in large quantities, they quickly move through the digestive tract, often causing diarrhea and abdominal cramping.

- This group includes *sorbitol, mannitol, maltitol,* and *xylitol.* Keep those "-itol" words in mind when you look at food labels when shopping. Foods in this category include avocados, plums, peaches, cauliflower, and some sugar-free or diet products.

As you might expect, some foods contain more than one FODMAP, making it difficult to group them in one category. These foods include apples, pears, watermelon, sweet corn, and coconut flour.

What Is the Low-FODMAP Diet?

The low-FODMAP diet is a two-phase process that allows those of us who follow it to identify our own personal triggers. The first phase is an elimination diet, which consists of completely avoiding foods that are high in FODMAPs. Experts recommend following the elimination phase for six to eight weeks, but you can start seeing results or improvements in just seven days. The second phase is a reintroduction process, which consists of adding FODMAPs back into the diet one group at a time, beginning with a small amount and then gradually increasing the amount of that food group.

THE ORIGINS OF THE LOW-FODMAP DIET

The acronym "FODMAP" was first used in 2005 by a group of Australian researchers at Monash University, who suggested that these types of carbohydrates are responsible for the symptoms experienced by IBS (irritable bowel syndrome) patients. They conducted a study looking at patients with IBS and fructose malabsorption, who restricted their intake of fructose, fructans, and in some cases polyols. The results showed that 74 percent of patients who followed the dietary restrictions had significant symptom improvement. Those who were even more compliant with the diet had better results. Since then, several studies have confirmed that restriction of FODMAPs helps improve symptoms in people who suffer from IBS.

It's important to go through the reintroduction process, since not all FODMAPs are triggers for all people who suffer from IBS. Given the restrictiveness of the diet, it's great to find out which FODMAPs your body can tolerate so you don't permanently give up foods unless you have to. For example, I'm able to tolerate honey, stone fruits, chickpeas (also known as garbanzo beans), coconut water, coconut milk, and dried fruits. Another thing to consider is that most high-FODMAP foods are rich in vitamins, minerals, antioxidants, and fiber. If you avoid them all for life, you can put yourself at risk of developing nutrient deficiencies. So if it's a food you can tolerate, there's no reason to avoid it.

The list of which foods to choose and which to lose can be confusing. I keep a copy of the chart on the next two pages on me at all times to help ease grocery shopping and dining out. Carry it with you so you can access it whenever you're unsure of a food and its FODMAP levels.

WHAT TO CHOOSE (LOW-FODMAP)

DAIRY & PROTEIN

All meats and seafood (beef, fish, poultry)

Almond milk

Coconut yogurt

Eggs

Hard cheeses (including Cheddar, Colby, feta, mozzarella, Parmesan, and Swiss)

Lactose-free dairy products

Lactose-free kefir

Rice milk

Tempeh

Tofu (soft or firm but not silken)

FRUITS

Blueberries

Cantaloupe

Clementines

Cranberries

Grapes

Honeydew melons

Kiwifruit

Oranges

Papayas

Pineapple

Raspberries

Rhubarb

Strawberries

VEGETABLES

Bamboo shoots

Bean sprouts

Carrots

Chives

Collard Greens

Cucumbers

Eggplant

Fennel leaves

Kale

Lettuce (all kinds)

Parsnips

Potatoes

Pickles

Radishes

Red bell peppers

Spinach

Summer squash

Tomatoes, common

Winter squash

Spaghetti squash

Swiss chard

Zucchini

GRAINS & STARCHES

Corn chips

Corn tortillas

Gluten-free white bread

Grits

Pasta made from corn, quinoa, or rice

Polenta

Popcorn

Quinoa

Rice (any variety)

Rice crackers

PULSES AND NUTS

Almond butter

Chia seeds

Flax seeds

Peanuts

Peanut butter

Pumpkin seeds (pepitas)

Sunflower seeds

PANTRY STAPLES

Avocado oil

Brown rice syrup

Butter

Cacao powder

Dark chocolate

Ghee

Gingerroot

Mayonnaise

Mustard

Olives

Olive oil

Raw sugar

Soy sauce

Stevia

BEVERAGES

Black coffee

Black, green, or white tea

Certain herbal teas (such as ginger and peppermint)

Cranberry juice

Gin

Vodka

Whiskey

Wine

WHAT TO LOSE (HIGH-FODMAP)

DAIRY & PROTEIN

Buttermilk

Condensed milk

Custard

Dry powdered milk

Evaporated milk

Frozen yogurt

Ice cream

Milk from cows, goats, and sheep

Soft, unripened cheeses (cream cheese, cottage cheese, mascarpone, ricotta)

Soy milk*

Yogurt

FRUITS

Apples (including apple juice, apple cider, and applesauce)

Apricots

Avocados

Blackberries

Cherries.

Dried fruits (including dried fruit juices)

Mangos

Nectarines

Peaches

Pears (including pear juice)

Pomegranate

Plums

Watermelon

VEGETABLES

Artichokes

Asparagus

Beets

Brussels sprouts

Cabbage (savoy)

Cauliflower

Garlic

Green peas

Leeks

Mushrooms

Onions

Pumpkin

Radicchio

Scallion bulbs

Shallots

Snow peas

Sugar snap peas

Sweet corn

GRAINS & STARCHES

Barley

Bread

Coconut flour

Couscous

Gnocchi (from wheat)

Oatmeal

Rye

Spelt

Wheat and derivatives

PULSES AND NUTS

Beans

Cashews

Chickpeas (garbanzo beans)

Veggie burgers (containing soy and beans)

Lentils

Pistachios

Silken tofu

PANTRY STAPLES

Agave nectar

Agave syrup

Crystalline fructose

High-fructose corn syrup

Honey

Molasses

Pancake syrup

BEVERAGES

Carob powder

Certain herbal teas (chamomile, fennel, oolong)

Chai

Eggnog

Rum

Strongly brewed teas (including kombucha)

Soft drinks (with high-fructose corn syrup)

* In the United States, soy milk products are commonly made from whole soybeans, which are high-FODMAP. However, soy milk made from soy protein is low-FODMAP.

Relief in Seven Days

As previously mentioned, most low-FODMAP diet plans recommend following a six- to eight-week strategy, but for anyone suffering from stomach discomfort, that can feel like a lifetime. Let me clarify: A seven-day plan does not mean that after those seven days you will be feeling 100 percent better. But it does allow for enough time to know if the diet may work for you. For me, it was a no-brainer to try it if there was any possibility it might work. I knew I couldn't feel any worse, so what was there to lose?

If you strictly follow the diet, you can expect to find a major reduction in symptoms like digestive discomfort, gas, bloating, diarrhea, and/or constipation. After the first few days, I noticed a major reduction in gas and bloating, which was a huge incentive for me to keep moving forward with the process. If after those first seven days, you've noticed a positive difference, I encourage you to continue avoiding all FODMAPs a little longer, to better understand how the diet works and what a low-FODMAP meal looks like for you.

Keep in mind that if you have constipation, it may take a little longer for these sugars to completely leave your body, which is why you may need to stick to the

WHY OUR BODIES NEED (SOME) FODMAPS

It can seem counterintuitive at first that healthy foods like apples, plums, asparagus, and cauliflower need to be initially eliminated from your diet. The low-FODMAP diet isn't really about "healthy" versus "unhealthy" or the endless battle of "good foods" versus "bad foods." It's about finding the foods that your body is unable to digest or absorb properly. Most people aren't reactive to every single FODMAP category, and high-FODMAP foods are often packed with vitamins and minerals important for the body, so it's crucial not to do a straight elimination of all the foods on the list forever. If you don't react to a particular FODMAP, you want to keep foods containing it in your diet in order to benefit from their healthy nutrients. (In fact, oligosaccharides like fructans and galactans have been shown to promote the growth of good bacteria like lactobacillus, so if you don't react to them, they may actually be good for your digestive health!)

Personally, I've figured out that I can eat stone fruits, honey, and chickpeas. On the other hand, I've tried many times to add lactose, onions, and garlic back into my diet with no luck. Like I said before, every person's digestive system is different!

first part of the diet longer; however, it's usually unnecessary to continue with these strict restrictions for longer than eight weeks. And if eight weeks seems impossible in the beginning, you'll be shocked at how easy it is to stick with it once you start noticing a difference in how you feel.

Are FODMAPs a Problem for You?

Many people come to the low-FODMAP diet after suffering from bloating, gas, abdominal pain/discomfort, diarrhea, or constipation for some time. Usually, these people are dealing with IBS, SIBO, IBD, and/or difficulty with gluten.

IBS: IBS stands for "irritable bowel syndrome." While it's estimated that 10 to 15 percent of US adults have IBS, only 5 to 7 percent have been diagnosed. IBS is more common in women and people under age 45. The diagnosis for IBS is more of an elimination process, since there is no specific test to make a diagnosis. Though we don't fully understand the causes, people who suffer from IBS have increased pain, discomfort, and bloating, because the bacteria in the intestines do more fermentation and produce more gas than is normal. Elimination of high-FODMAP foods helps to reduce gas production, bloating, and changes in bowel movements.

SIBO: SIBO stands for "small intestinal bacteria overgrowth." People who suffer from IBS have higher rates of SIBO. Symptoms can vary from mild to severe bloating, increased belching, chronic diarrhea, and, in severe cases, weight loss and malabsorption. There are several ways to diagnose SIBO, but the most widely used are the hydrogen and methane breath tests. Treatment may include a course of antibiotics, and some practitioners recommend a low-FODMAP diet because it limits the bacteria's food source and thus their growth. However, more studies are needed to prove that a low-FODMAP diet really works for SIBO.

IBD: IBD stands for "inflammatory bowel disease," and there is growing evidence that a low-FODMAP diet can help manage symptoms for patients with this disorder. IBD refers to chronic inflammation of all or part of the digestive tract and more specifically includes Crohn's disease (which primarily affects the small intestine) and ulcerative colitis (which affects the colon and rectum). According to the Crohn's & Colitis Foundation, 1.6 million Americans currently suffer from this disease, and 70,000 new cases of IBD are diagnosed each year. A study by Dr. Richard Gearry and colleagues published in 2009 included 52 patients with active Crohn's disease and 20 with active ulcerative colitis. All were instructed by a registered dietitian on a low-FODMAP diet. The results showed that 70 percent of patients who followed the low-FODMAP diet had a greater improvement in abdominal pain, bloating, and diarrhea.

GLUTEN: Gluten-related disorders include celiac disease, which is an autoimmune condition, and gluten intolerance or sensitivity, among others. Celiac disease is an immune reaction triggered when a person eats gluten. It leads to damage to the small-intestinal lining, which can lead to symptoms like diarrhea, bloating, gas, and malabsorption. The diagnosis of celiac disease can be challenging; it can include a blood test that must be done while you're still eating gluten and/or an endoscopy to look at the lining of your small intestine and take a small sample of intestinal tissue to see if there has been any damage. It has been estimated that 1 in 141 Americans suffer from celiac disease, but many may have not been diagnosed yet. People who have tested negative for celiac disease but have symptoms when eating gluten are diagnosed with a gluten intolerance. Currently, there is no specific test to diagnose a gluten intolerance or sensitivity. There are people who may feel some improvement while following a gluten-free diet but continue to experience some gas, bloating, abdominal pain, diarrhea, and/or constipation. A low-FODMAP diet would help identify if there are any additional intolerances to foods. Though gluten is not a FODMAP, a low-FODMAP diet restricts wheat, barley, and rye, which all contain gluten.

The common themes of all the above-mentioned health conditions are bloating, gas, abdominal pain/discomfort, diarrhea, and/or constipation. A temporary FODMAP elimination can help ease all these symptoms; however, it's important to ask your health-care provider before starting a new diet.

You Have Nothing to Lose— Except Discomfort

I know it can feel overwhelming at first to wrap your head around FODMAPs while simultaneously making a major change to your diet. Think back to when I asked you how you were initially feeling. I'm guessing you weren't feeling your best. So what do you have to lose: bloating, gas, and stomach pain? I'd gladly lose those any day!

FIBER AND FODMAPS

There are many ways to categorize fiber: short or long; soluble or insoluble; highly fermentable; slowly fermentable; or nonfermentable. For those with IBS, the main fiber types that cause symptoms are those that are short in size, soluble, and moderately to highly fermentable. Foods that contain these types of fiber include apples, beans, lentils, and wheat bran, all of which should be avoided.

If you have constipation and need to take a fiber supplement while on a low-FODMAP diet, consider a fiber that is nonfermentable, like cellulose or methylcellulose. Psyllium, which is moderately fermentable, has also worked for some people with IBS. Of course, always discuss dietary changes with your health-care provider first.

I remember having those same overwhelming emotions when I first started the low-FODMAP diet, but even more vividly, I remember doing a little dance when my digestive symptoms began to dissipate. There is so much to gain by trying this plan. Give it an honest seven days to see how much better you can feel.

The biggest upside with the low-FODMAP diet is that the elimination of all high-FODMAP foods is usually not a lifelong recommendation. Instead, it's a process to figure out what foods are triggers for you. In just seven days, you can vastly reduce or eliminate the bloating, gas, cramping, diarrhea, and constipation that you, like I once was, are accustomed to suffering from.

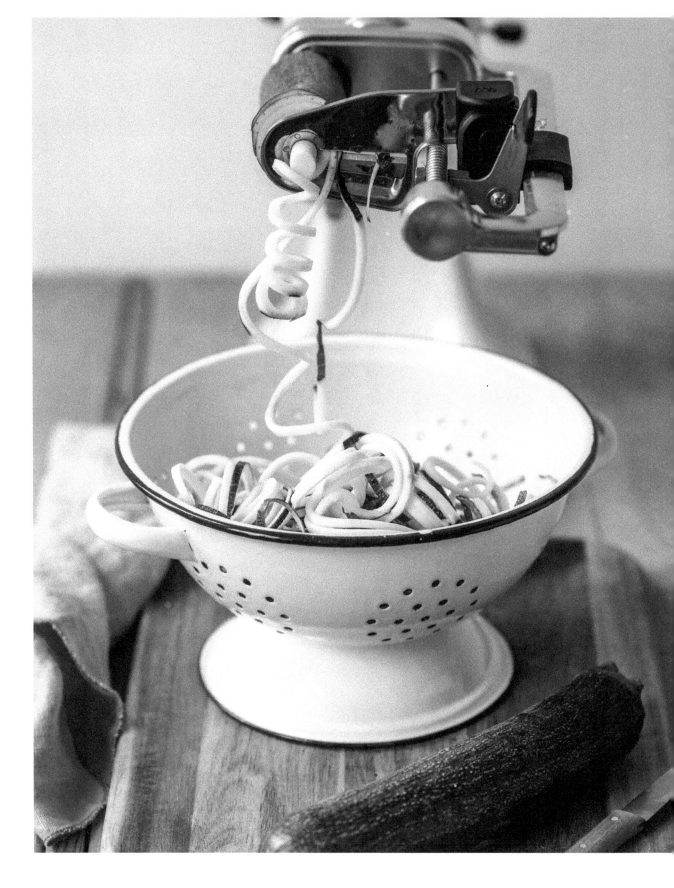

Chapter 2

The Low-FODMAP Diet in Five Steps

For me, breaking down any daunting new challenge into doable steps makes it much more manageable, whether it's a work assignment, planning a wedding, or, in this case, a new diet. I've come up with five straightforward steps for approaching a low-FODMAP diet. It's true, these are not "official" steps, but this is what I did as I transitioned to a low-FODMAP diet. The step-by-step approach helped make it a little less intimidating and gave me confidence that I could really do this.

Organize Your Pantry

If you're anything like me, after reviewing the list of high- and low-FODMAP foods, your first instinct might be to throw out anything and everything that falls into the high-FODMAP category. Let me stop you and instead suggest you put these items on a different shelf in the pantry or store them in a box so you know that they're off-limits while you're in the elimination phase. Every one of us tolerates certain high-FODMAP foods differently, and you may find that you can still enjoy some of these foods once you try reintroducing them into your diet.

THE GOOD STUFF

Even though the low-FODMAP diet is restrictive, there are still lots of foods that are low in FODMAPs and can be part of a healthy lifestyle. For instance, eggs, lean meats, lactose-free dairy, brown rice, corn, and potatoes are all allowed. For a detailed list of low-FODMAP pantry staples, see page 8 in chapter 1.

It can be a challenge to find brands that have low-FODMAP products, but they are out there. Here are a few of my favorite low-FODMAP products. Note that while I list them by brand, not all products made by these brands are low-FODMAP.

- **88 ACRES:** Their Chocolate & Sea Salt bar, "Seednola" (granola made with seeds), and seed butters are all FODMAP-safe.
- **GLUTINO:** Their pretzels are a great low-FODMAP snack to have on hand. This brand is completely gluten-free (which means no high-FODMAP wheat) and easy to find in most grocery stores.
- **JOVIAL:** I love their brown-rice pastas. This brand is also completely gluten-free and has a wide range of FODMAP-safe products available.

A food that I love to recommend when starting your road to good digestive health is kefir, which is a cultured milk that contains natural probiotics (good bacteria for your gut). Lifeway's plain kefir is 99 percent lactose-free, has no added sugars, and contains 12 live active cultures of probiotics.

THE NOT-NOW STUFF

So, what to do with all the high-FODMAP foods that you've set aside? In some cases, you may be able to add them back into your diet shortly after the elimination period, which is why I suggested storing them away for the short term. In general,

LOW-FODMAP FOR VEGETARIANS

The low-FODMAP diet is compatible with a vegetarian lifestyle with simple swaps you can adapt into the meal plan. Most vegetarian diets revolve around legumes and vegetables, which, unfortunately, are often high-FODMAP. Make sure to eliminate these completely for the duration of the seven days and reintroduce them back in one at a time once you're symptom-free to make sure they're not the source of your discomfort. Through the reintroduction process, you'll find out if you can handle a smaller serving size of high-FODMAP foods and be just fine. For example, I've been able to add chickpeas back into my diet.

Unfortunately, vegan considerations are more involved and beyond the scope of this book. I recommend you check out *Low-FODMAP and Vegan* by Jo Stepaniak if you eat a plant-based diet and want to do a low-FODMAP elimination diet as well.

One of the main concerns for vegetarians is the restriction of pulses, which is a main source of protein and fiber. Low-FODMAP vegetarian proteins that aren't legumes include:

- Eggs
- Lactose-free and nondairy milks and yogurts
- Firm tofu (avoid silken tofu) and tempeh
- Grains like quinoa, buckwheat, polenta, and steel-cut oats (mind serving sizes)
- Certain nuts and seeds in recommended serving sizes
- Canned lentils*

Tests show that canned lentils have a lower FODMAP count than soaked pulses. You can initially try a ½-cup serving of canned lentils, but make sure they don't contain garlic or onions.

packaged and prepared foods have many hidden FODMAP ingredients. If you're not sure which to put aside, review the ingredient lists for any of these words: high-fructose corn syrup, onion powder, garlic powder, agave syrup, honey, inulin, chicory root, and sugar alcohols (sorbitol, mannitol, maltitol, xylitol, and isomalt).

If space is tight and you'd rather not keep these tempting, off-limits products around, consider donating them to a homeless shelter or sharing them with family members and friends (who don't have IBS, of course!).

Plan Your Meals

I cannot stress enough the importance of having a meal plan when undertaking an elimination diet for the first time. This will ease the stress and anxiety of having to figure out what to eat, particularly when you're short on time and hungry. When you have a meal plan, everything is already planned and ready for you to follow—no stress!

I plan my meals every weekend, taking some time on Saturday to decide which meals I'd like to have during the week. I consider any plans I already have for eating out, make sure I include a snack or two to prepare, plan mostly familiar meals I know I can pull off quickly, and sometimes add a new meal in for variety.

The meal plan included in this book consists of three meals plus two snacks per day, with meal-prep guidelines and a comprehensive shopping list for the week.

Taking the "wing it" approach often leads to bad choices at worst or additional trips to the grocery store at best. Like my parents used to say, the more prepared you are, the better the outcome.

CUSTOMIZING YOUR MEAL PLANS

Chapter 3 of this book includes a one-week meal plan that you can extend and reuse as many times as you would like. Feel free to swap out the meal plan with the recipes from part 2 of the book to create your own customized plan. All recipes in the book will work for the low-FODMAP diet.

Step 3

Buy and Prep Food

With your meal plan set, it's time to go grocery shopping. I like exploring local weekend farmers' markets. They have the freshest produce available, plus there's no need to read labels when purchasing fresh fruits and vegetables. Wherever you shop, bring your quick reference list for low-FODMAP fruits and vegetables, or download the Monash University app (see page 143).

FOOD SHOPPING

Food shopping in the afternoon or evening on Sunday can be extremely stressful. I prefer to do my shopping first thing in the morning, or even on Saturday. I don't want to be rushed or feel anxious when I'm shopping for food. For your first forays into low-FODMAP grocery shopping, give yourself extra time to review labels and explore foods that are naturally low-FODMAP.

The Basics

Before beginning the elimination diet, there are some low-FODMAP basics you can stock up on (or review your pantry to see if you already have them). They include:

- Water and tea (green, black, rooibos, ginger, and peppermint).
- Sea salt, black pepper, and fresh or dried herbs like oregano, thyme, parsley, chili powder, and cumin. For some people with IBS, black pepper, chili powder, and paprika can be irritating. Feel free to replace them with cilantro, parsley, marjoram, rosemary, or bay leaves.
- Garlic-infused extra-virgin olive oil.
- Mayonnaise, mustard (garlic- and onion-free), and soy sauce.
- Beef, chicken, and vegetable broths, as well as bone broth. Just make sure these store-bought products do not contain garlic or onion.
- Nuts and seeds such as pecans, walnuts, almonds, pumpkin seeds, and sunflower seeds. (Make sure to refer to the recommended servings.)

Animal Protein

The low-FODMAP diet does not restrict animal proteins, fish, or eggs. I do advise you to watch your intake of pork, beef, and other red meats, as they can be hard for the stomach to digest properly. In fact, I don't include any recipes with pork or beef in this book. Choose lean meats and wild-caught fish and seafood instead.

Produce

This is when carrying the FODMAP reference chart (see page 8) around with you comes in handy. Stick to fruits and vegetables like unripe bananas, strawberries, oranges, pineapple, green beans, spinach, and carrots, which are all low-FODMAP. Choose fruits and vegetables of multiple colors; variety is best!

A word about bananas: This fruit has been retested by the FODMAP researchers at Monash University and found to be higher in fructans when ripe. If you're going to include bananas in your low-FODMAP diet and/or recipe, choose unripe bananas or limit your intake to one-third of a medium-ripe banana.

FINDING FODMAPS IN INGREDIENT LISTS

It might take an extra few seconds to read ingredient labels while grocery shopping to look for hidden FODMAPs in foods, but it's worth the effort. In no time, you'll be an expert at spotting and avoiding these triggers. The keywords to focus on are: high-fructose corn syrup, onion powder, garlic powder, agave syrup, molasses, honey, inulin, chicory root, and sugar alcohols (sorbitol, mannitol, malt-itol, xylitol, and isomalt). Unfortunately, these are found in most packaged foods. Be aware that even if a package says "healthy" or "gluten-free," the food inside can still be high-FODMAP. Be particularly suspicious if a package says "sugar-free"—that often means it's sweetened with sugar alcohols instead.

Ingredients are listed on a label in order of quantity, from most to least. If one or more of these keywords is listed near the top of the ingredient list, that means the quantity of that item is much higher than if it were listed near the bottom.

Look at the two ingredient lists in the next column. I've highlighted the high-FODMAP ingredients.

INGREDIENTS: Tomato purée (water, tomato paste), vegetable oil (contains one or more of the following: soybean oil, corn oil), **high-fructose corn syrup**, salt, **dried onions**, extra-virgin olive oil, Romano cheese (cow's milk, cheese cultures, salt, enzymes), spices, natural flavor.

INGREDIENTS: Water, soybean oil, distilled vinegar, sugar, salt, contains 2% or less of each of the following: **garlic***, **onion***, red bell peppers*, xanthan gum, maltodextrin (corn), spices, autolyzed yeast extract, calcium disodium EDTA (used to protect quality), natural flavor, lemon-juice concentrate, caramel color, annatto extract (color). *Dried. Gluten-free.

There are some additional sneaky ingredients that you'll want to keep an eye out for, including:

- All-purpose flour: Contains wheat.

- Dry milk solids or whey protein: Contains lactose.

Dairy

Lactose, a naturally occurring sugar component in dairy, is not permitted on the low-FODMAP diet—but be mindful that there is a difference between "lactose-free" and "dairy-free," and some dairy products can be lactose-free. Lactose-free milk and yogurt and hard/aged cheeses are examples of dairy allowed on the low-FODMAP diet. Nut- and plant-based milks, like almond and coconut milk, are also acceptable substitutes for regular milk.

Fats and Oils

We all need healthy fats and oils to support our metabolism, immunity, and general body health. Oils don't contain carbohydrates, which means they don't contain FODMAPs. Olive oil, avocado oil, flaxseed oil, and other oils are FODMAP safe.

FOOD PREP

I am a big proponent of preparing food ahead of time, as it makes for a much more pleasant diet experience. It has now become second nature for me to do meal prep on Sundays for the upcoming week. My breakfasts, snacks, and other miscellaneous items are prepped, chopped, and cooked so I can grab and go during the week. I'm all about simple, easy, and fast.

Five Tips for Successful Meal Prepping:

1. **Sort your ingredients.** Have all ingredients on the counter before beginning to prep and cook.

2. **Buy precut vegetables if necessary.** I buy these for vegetables that are time consuming to prep, like acorn squash.

3. **Set aside one day a week.** When possible, commit to one day a week on which you can prep, chop, and cook. It's a huge time-saver for the rest of the week.

4. **Clean as you go.** The process feels so much easier when you're not facing a sink full of dishes at the end.

5. **Use storage containers.** Store prepared foods in airtight containers or zip-top plastic bags to preserve all the hard work you just did. Most items will keep in the refrigerator for a week.

Step 4
Do the Diet

This diet has worked for so many people, myself included, and it shouldn't take multiple weeks to feel relief. This book has you start with just one week of the elimination diet to make it more approachable. The hardest part is starting, but once you have your meal plan and food prep taken care of, you're ready to go.

If you see positive results from the first week, I highly recommend you continue on and do another full week. Don't focus on how long you have to be on the diet before deciding to reintroduce a high-FODMAP food. Take it a week at a time and evaluate where you are on your road to feeling better after each week. The success of the diet lies in two parts: strictly following the elimination diet, and tracking your symptoms. If you're wondering what will happen if you don't follow the diet strictly, see page 43.

SYMPTOM TRACKING

Tracking your symptoms is a vital part of the seven-day elimination plan. It's important to note how you feel before beginning the seven days, and to track your symptoms as you go forward. That way you'll have a reference for which foods you're more sensitive to and which ones you had no reaction to. Plus, there's nothing more rewarding than seeing progress in terms of your health—it's a great reminder that all your hard work does pay off.

ELIMINATION DIET SYMPTOM TRACKER

Use this page to track symptoms each day during the elimination diet. You can also download the form from callistomediabooks.com/lowfodmapforbeginners. If you repeat the diet after the first week, continue to track symptoms, which will be especially encouraging as they disappear.

DAY	SYMPTOMS
1	
2	
3	
4	
5	
6	
7	

Reintroduce FODMAPs

Once you've finished your FODMAP-free week (or weeks), you can start doing "food challenges" to reintroduce each type of FODMAP back into your diet, one by one. The goal of a food challenge is to add moderate- or high-FODMAP foods back into your diet while still having positive results (that is, no symptoms or a reduction of symptoms). The overarching purpose of the elimination diet is not to permanently remove foods from your diet but rather to add back as many of your favorite FODMAP foods as possible, without the symptoms.

Foods should be reintroduced one group at a time—just fructose, then just lactose, and so forth. There is no one recommended order to be followed. If you're a dairy lover, lactose is one of the easiest groups to reintroduce to determine if you have a lactose intolerance. Foods that include more than one FODMAP—such as apples, which have fructose and polyols—can be a little more difficult. If you have symptoms after eating one, it's hard to know which FODMAP group caused the reaction. For this reason, chapter 4 offers more guidance on careful reintroductions.

Common Challenges and Mistakes

Universally, there are common challenges and mistakes many people face when beginning the low-FODMAP diet. Here I'll list several of these, followed by my tips for addressing them.

THERE'S NO EASY WAY TO REMEMBER WHICH FOODS ARE LOW-FODMAP. This is where the chart in chapter 1 comes in handy as a quick reference guide (see page 8), as does the Monash University Low-FODMAP Diet app.

DON'T EAT SO MUCH OF A MODERATE-FODMAP FOOD THAT IT BECOMES A HIGH-FODMAP FOOD. Portion size is just as important as what you eat. If you eat a large amount of a relatively moderate-FODMAP food, the overall FODMAP count can start to get big. You can eat as many different low-FODMAP foods as you like but be careful with those that have a recommended portion size.

DIFFERENT FODMAP FOOD LISTS SAY DIFFERENT THINGS. There are a lot of inconsistencies out there. Foods are being tested and retested at Australia's Monash

PORTION IS KEY

Those of us who commit to eating low-FODMAP for any period of time need to pay attention to the portion sizes of some foods within a meal. We must measure what we eat, particularly fruits. All fruits have fructose, but if you stick to the recommended serving size, you probably won't ingest enough of it to cause a reaction. As a general guideline, you can eat two servings of low-FODMAP fruits and five servings of low-FODMAP vegetables per day.

The chart on page 27 lists specific portions sizes to follow for low- and moderate-FODMAP foods. Keep in mind that these portions are per meal, assuming meals are eaten three hours apart, not total for the day. For example, the recommended portion size for green bell peppers is ½ cup, so you can have ½ cup of green bell peppers in your salad at lunch and another ½ cup serving at dinner. You'll still be safe portion-wise, because you're eating the portion in two different meals. Some of the portions may seem small, but they're recommended based on research and testing. Stick to the suggested serving size for the first week until you challenge (that is, reintroduce) a higher amount at a later date.

Also note that there is not one generic serving size for all fruits, all vegetables, all dairy products, etc. The correct portion amount varies for each individual food. This is important to adhere to and note while you track your symptoms.

University for FODMAP content, but imagine how many different foods exist in the world. Some foods thought to be low-FODMAP have been found to be high-FODMAP, and vice versa. The chapter 1 chart (see page 8) is a good first step. The Monash University Low-FODMAP Diet app includes updates on newly tested foods and portion sizes.

SOMETIMES THE DIET SEEMS TOO HARD, BUT CONTINUING IS WORTH IT. Feeling discouraged and overwhelmed happens to the best of us. I highly recommend joining online FODMAP communities for support. It's a great way to be part of a community that understands what you've gone through in the past and what you're currently experiencing. A few of my favorite Facebook groups are Fodmap For Your Health, Low FODMAP Diet and IBS, and IBS & The Low FODMAP Diet.

DON'T DESPAIR IF SOME OF YOUR FAVORITE FOODS ARE HIGH-FODMAP. The goal of the elimination diet is to be able to reintroduce high-FODMAP foods back into your diet. If you reintroduce them too quickly and have an adverse reaction, don't beat yourself up. Your body is just letting you know it's not ready for those foods yet. Just start over and stick to the plan as best you can.

Remember to Support Yourself

It's natural to feel overwhelmed by the idea of eliminating so many foods and planning your meals. Even the thought of undertaking such a big change can be frightening. You've already taken one of the biggest steps by buying this book. Often we spend so much energy and time thinking about how difficult change can be rather than thinking of all the benefits we can gain by just trying. It's so important to love and take care of yourself. Keep in mind that there's a bigger purpose past the seven-day elimination diet, which includes a general improvement of your health. You've got this!

Here are five practical, concrete tips to help you feel less alone, stay motivated, and cultivate greater compassion for yourself.

Join an online FODMAP community or Facebook group. This is a great way to ask questions, hear success stories, and receive support. On Facebook, these are the three groups I love:

- Fodmap For Your Health
- Low FODMAP Diet and IBS
- IBS & The Low FODMAP Diet

Keep a journal tracking your progress and emotions. It's a tangible way to see improvements within yourself. Here are some of my specific recommendations.

- Reward yourself after the first seven days. It can be something small like treating yourself to a movie or something bigger like going to the spa.
- Involve your family and friends in the process. Encouragement from those you love helps set you up for success.
- Exercise every day, even if it's just a walk around the block. The increase of endorphins you get from exercising is well worth it and will help you keep a positive attitude.

RECOMMENDED PORTION SIZES FOR
LOW-FODMAP AND MODERATE-FODMAP FOODS

Here you'll find recommended portion sizes for a variety of common low- and moderate-FODMAP foods, as outlined by Monash University researchers. Make sure to pay attention to serving sizes for moderate-FODMAP foods, just as you would with high-FODMAP items.

So much can be gained in your meals and snacks by adding some of these moderate foods back in if you're able to tolerate them. If you do not see a food here that is on the list of low-FODMAP foods to choose on page 8, you can assume it is safe to eat in larger quantities.

DAIRY & PROTEIN	PORTION
Cheddar cheese	1 ounce
Colby cheese	1 ounce
Feta cheese	1 ounce
Half-and-half	2 tbsps
Mozzarella cheese	1 ounce
Parmesan cheese (hard)	1 ounce
Sour cream	2 tbsps
Soy milk (made from soy protein)	1 cup
Swiss cheese	1 ounce

FRUITS	PORTION
Avocado	⅛ of whole
Banana (unripe)	1 (medium)
Blueberries	½ cup
Cantaloupe	½ cup
Clementine	1 (medium)
Cranberries (raw)	½ cup
Coconut	½ cup
Grapes	½ cup
Honeydew melon	½ cup
Kiwi	1 (medium)
Orange	1 (small)
Papaya	½ cup
Pineapple	½ cup
Raspberries	½ cup
Rhubarb	½ cup
Strawberries	½ cup

VEGETABLES	PORTION
Broccoli	1 cup
Bok choy	1 cup
Butternut squash	¼ cup
Fennel bulb	½ cup
Green bell pepper	½ cup
Green beans	12
Rutabaga	½ cup
Snow peas	5 pods
Sweet potato	½ cup
Tomatoes, cherry	4
Tomato, Roma	1 (small)
Turnip	½ cup

GRAINS & STARCHES	PORTION
Amaranth	¼ cup
Oats	½ cup

PULSES AND NUTS	PORTION
Almonds	2 tbsps/10 nuts
Canned chickpeas	¼ cup
Canned lentils	½ cup
Hazelnuts	2 tbsps/10 nuts
Pecans	2 tbsps/10 nuts

PANTRY STAPLES	PORTION
Coconut milk (canned)	⅓ cup
Maple syrup	1 tbsp

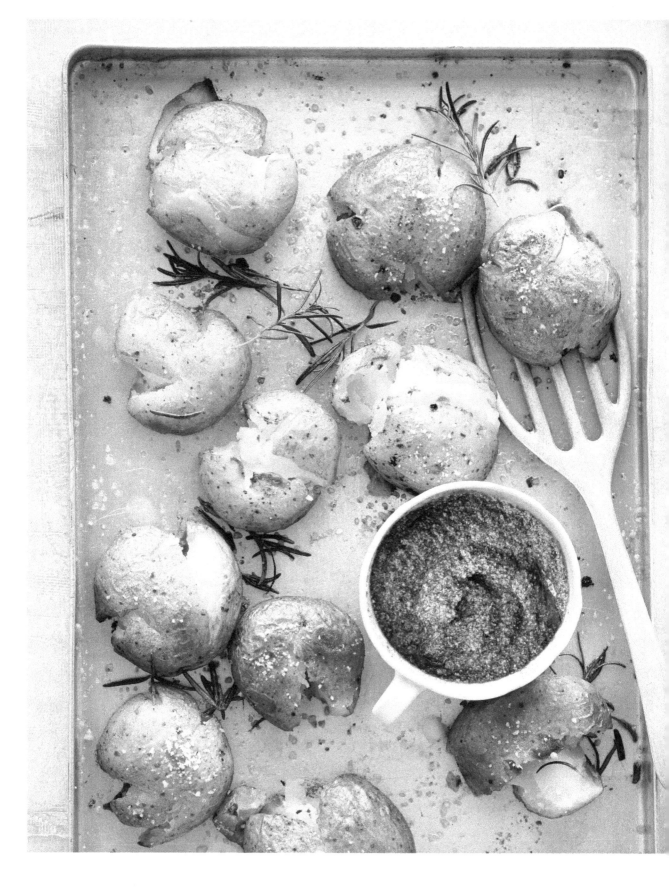

Your Seven-Day Elimination Diet

This book offers a seven-day elimination diet, and all recipes are gluten-free and low-FODMAP. Feel free to explore the recipes and swap some out if you have a preference for other low-FODMAP recipes. While the elimination diet is for omnivores, there are a number of vegetarian and vegan recipes in part 2 of the book to swap out for recipes that include meat. Just make sure you reflect any recipe changes in the shopping list included in this chapter. The seven-day meal plan, shopping list, and recipe list in this chapter are what you can follow for the entire week. Trust me when I say doing this will make the week ahead so much easier and less stressful.

Left: Smashed Potatoes (page 65)

This meal plan does include make-ahead recipes as well as suggestions to repurpose the leftovers. One of the snacks on the meal plan involves baking, but otherwise the snacks are generally no-cook and no-fuss. To make things simpler, there are no desserts on the meal plan, but if you, like me, have a major sweet tooth, chapter 10 does include sweet snacks and desserts you can make. If you choose to make a dessert, be sure to add those ingredients to the shopping list. If you're looking for the easiest dessert recipe ever, try my Banana Ice Cream (page 118).

Setting Expectations

It's always important to set realistic expectations before starting this diet. The results and symptom relief I've had may differ from yours. For me, the first thing I noticed was being hungrier than usual, and I've heard many others say the same. One of the reasons why is probably that I eliminated many prepackaged foods that contained FODMAP triggers. It does take a little time for your body to adjust to the change, which is completely normal. I noticed almost immediately the reduction of bloating and gas, which was the biggest encouragement for me in continuing with the elimination diet.

Per IBSdiets.org, about 85 percent of patients find relief when following the low-FODMAP diet, but there are still 15 percent of people who don't. This could be for a number of reasons, including not being sensitive to FODMAPs (yay for you!), sucrase deficiency, or other food sensitivities or intolerances. Those who struggle to follow the elimination process correctly may also fail to find relief.

Preparation here pays off. The less you have to fuss and cook during the week, the more likely you'll be able to stick to the plan. (See page 35 for a prep guide.)

This meal plan consists of three meals and two snacks per day for Monday through Sunday. I'm a big proponent of making breakfast, lunch, and dinner as easy as possible, which for me involves prepping ingredients and making some dishes ahead the weekend before, then using them throughout the week.

THE ELIMINATION DIET

	BREAKFAST	SNACK	LUNCH	SNACK	DINNER
M	Green Monster Smoothie (p. 56)	⅓ unripe banana with 1 tablespoon natural peanut butter	Deli-meat sandwich on gluten-free bread with baby carrots and tortilla	Banana-Bread Muffins (p. 113)	Chicken Piccata with gluten-free pasta (p. 102)
T	Strawberry Split Smoothie (p. 57)	Banana-Bread Muffins (p. 113)	Leftover Chicken Piccata with gluten-free pasta (p. 102)	Peanut-Butter Energy Balls (p. 112)	Turkey Tacos and a Basic Salad (pp. 108, 70)
W	Baked Vegetable Egg Muffins (p. 52)	Peanut-Butter Energy Balls (p. 112)	Leftover Turkey Tacos over salad (p. 108)	Baby carrots, cucumbers, and Roasted Eggplant Dip (p. 117)	Greek Chicken Kebabs, Traditional Greek Salad, and brown rice (pp. 100, 72)
T	2 scrambled eggs on corn tortillas	1 orange	Leftover Greek Chicken Kebabs, Traditional Greek Salad, and Roasted Eggplant Dip (pp. 100, 72, 117)	Peanut-Butter Energy Balls (p. 112)	Cornmeal-Crusted Fish Tacos with Coleslaw (p. 92)
F	Baked Vegetable Egg Muffins (p. 52)	Peanut-Butter Energy Balls (p. 112)	Traditional Greek Salad (p. 72)	Baby carrots, cucumbers, and Roasted Eggplant Dip (p. 117)	Pasta with Fresh Basil, Tomato, and Zucchini (p. 80)
S	Easy French Toast (p. 49)	1 orange	2 corn tortilla deli wraps	Baby carrots, cucumbers, and Roasted Eggplant Dip (p. 117)	Dad's Easy Grilled Chicken, Grilled Peppers, Zucchini, and Carrots, and brown rice (pp. 105, 64)
S	Banana Pancakes (p. 48)	½ cup strawberries	Deli-meat sandwich on gluten-free bread with baby carrots and tortilla	Peanut-Butter Energy Balls (p. 112)	Baked Salmon with Smashed Potatoes and leftover Grilled Peppers, Zucchini, and Carrots (pp. 87, 65, 64)

Shopping List

The best way to be prepared and lower your stress level about taking on this seven-day elimination diet is to know what you're shopping for. Below is the shopping list for all the meals for the week. If you've swapped out any of the recipes for something else, be sure to adjust the shopping list.

CANNED AND BOTTLED ITEMS

- Capers, brined
- Maple syrup
- Peanut butter, all-natural
- Oil, coconut
- Vinegar, white wine
- Wine, white

DAIRY, EGGS, POULTRY, AND FISH

- Butter, unsalted
- Chicken breasts, boneless, skinless (6 [4 ounces each])
- Cod fillets (2 pounds)
- Eggs, large (16)
- Feta cheese crumbles
- Milk, lactose-free or nondairy
- Salmon fillets (12 ounces)
- Turkey, all-natural deli (½ pound)
- Turkey, ground (1 pound)

PANTRY ITEMS

- Nonstick cooking spray
- Baking soda
- Chili powder
- Cinnamon, ground
- Cornstarch, for dredging
- Cumin, dried
- Dijon mustard
- Oil, extra-virgin olive
- Oregano, dried
- Parsley, dried
- Peppercorns, black
- Salt, sea
- Sugar, raw (¾ cup)
- Vanilla extract
- Vinegar, balsamic

PRODUCE

- Arugula (1 [1-pound] bag)
- Bananas (7)
- Basil, fresh (1 bunch)
- Bell pepper, green (1)
- Bell peppers, mini
  (1 [1-pound] bag)
- Bell pepper, red (1)
- Bell pepper, yellow (1)
- Blueberries (½ cup)
- Cabbage, shredded (4 cups)
- Carrots (6)
- Carrots, baby (1 [1-pound] bag)
- Cucumbers (2)
- Eggplant (1)
- Lemons (3)
- Limes (2)
- Oranges (2)
- Parsley, fresh (1 bunch)
- Pineapple, frozen (½ cup)
- Potatoes, Yukon gold (6)
- Rosemary, fresh (2 sprigs)
- Salad leaves (1 pound)
- Scallions (1 tablespoon)
- Spinach (1½ cups)
- Strawberries (1 [1-pound] container)
- Tomatoes, cherry (1 [10½-ounce] container)
- Tomatoes, medium (5)
- Zucchini (4)

OTHER*

- Bread, gluten-free (8 slices)
- Chia seeds (3 tablespoons)
- Chocolate chips, dark
  (2 tablespoons)
- Cornmeal (½ cup)
- Flour, brown rice (1 tablespoon)
- Oats, old-fashioned (3½ cups)
- Pasta, gluten-free
  (2 [1-pound] boxes)
- Pumpkin seeds (¼ cup)
- Rice, brown (2 cups)
- Tortilla chips (1 [8-ounce] bag)
- Tortillas, corn (12)
- Vinegar, apple cider (½ teaspoon)
- Walnuts, chopped (½ cup)

* Before buying several of the products in this category—specifically bread, chocolate chips, pasta, tortilla chips, and tortillas—review package ingredients lists to ensure that they are low-FODMAP.

Recipes

BREAKFAST

- Green Monster Smoothie, page 56
- Strawberry Split Smoothie, page 57
- Baked Vegetable Egg Muffins, page 52
- Easy French Toast, page 49
- Banana Pancakes, page 48

SALAD AND VEGETABLES

- The Basic Salad, page 70
- Traditional Greek Salad, page 72
- Grilled Peppers, Zucchini, and Carrots, page 64
- Smashed Potatoes, page 65

DINNER

- Chicken Piccata, page 102
- Turkey Tacos, page 108
- Greek Chicken Kebabs, page 100
- Cornmeal-Crusted Fish Tacos with Coleslaw, page 92
- Pasta with Fresh Basil, Tomato, and Zucchini, page 80
- Dad's Easy Grilled Chicken, page 105
- Baked Salmon, page 87

SNACKS

- Peanut-Butter Energy Balls, page 112
- Banana-Bread Muffins, page 113
- Roasted Eggplant Dip, page 117

Prep Guide

The more prepared you are when you start anything new, the better the outcome. That's surely the case here as well. Plus prepping ahead of time has really become an enjoyable part of my Sunday routine.

WASH AND CUT

- Cucumbers: peel and dice 1 cucumber, slice 1 cucumber
- Scallion: chop
- Tomatoes: dice 4 tomatoes
- Mini bell peppers, dice
- Red bell pepper: cut into chunks

- Yellow bell pepper: cut into chunks
- Zucchini: cut 2 into thick rounds, dice 1
- Carrots: cut into thick rounds

COOK AND STORE

- Baked Vegetable Egg Muffins, page 52
- Banana-Bread Muffins, page 113

- Brown rice: 2 cups cooked
- Peanut-Butter Energy Balls, page 112

MAKE AHEAD

- Basic Vinaigrette, page 130
- Roasted Eggplant Dip, page 117

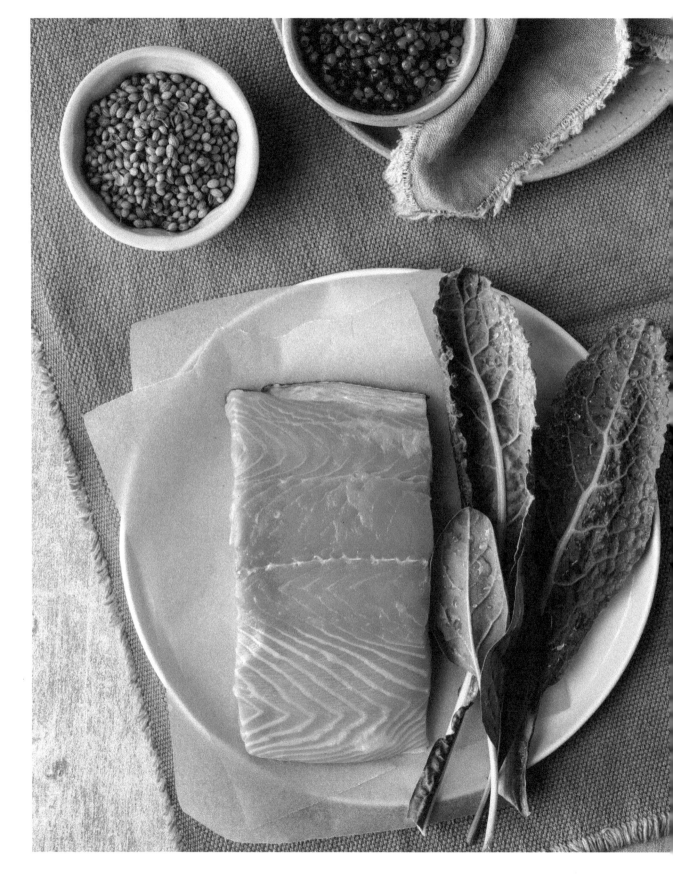

Chapter 4

Life After the Elimination Diet

Even if you haven't done the diet yet, you might be curious to know more about what happens after you do it. Although I had positive results during the elimination stage, I was nervous to start reintroducing high-FODMAP foods. Remember, the goal of this diet is not to remove all high-FODMAP foods completely from your diet but rather to exclude only the ones you can't tolerate. I encourage you to keep with the low-FODMAP elimination diet for another week or two and try a few other recipes from this book each week. Keep in mind that you may not want to start the reintroduction (or challenge) phase until you have achieved a significant improvement or complete resolution of symptoms. After you complete the food challenges, the last phase is your long-term low-FODMAP diet and your roadmap to staying symptom-free.

Reintroducing FODMAPs

There's no one right process to follow when reintroducing FODMAPs. Here are some general guidelines and things to keep in mind when starting the reintroduction phase.

- When testing a new food group, always begin with a very small portion size.
- If you didn't have any bad symptoms or reactions with a small portion, the next day you can increase or double the amount.
- If you had symptoms when challenging a food, stop testing and go back to the elimination diet for five to seven days to cleanse your system. Remember, you want to be symptom-free before challenging foods; otherwise you can get mixed or inaccurate results.
- Test one group at a time to clearly know which groups are a trigger for you. In other words, do not test dairy (lactose) and honey (fructose) at the same time.
- Keep a food diary and/or symptom tracker to stay on top of your results.

Lactose is the easiest group to reintroduce, since most dairy products don't contain other FODMAPs in addition to lactose. If you get symptoms from eating, say, an apple, you can't be sure if it's because of the fructose or the polyols, but the only FODMAP in milk is lactose, so you can easily determine whether you react to it or not. You can reintroduce this group first if you wish. Remember to start with a small portion and then gradually increase until you've reached the amount you were previously eating.

REINTRODUCING FOODS WITH MORE THAN ONE FODMAP

The presence of two or more FODMAPs in a food means there's a higher chance it will produce symptoms, so you have to test them with caution. A few examples include:

- apples (fructose and polyols)
- sweet corn (galactans and polyols)
- mushrooms (fructans and polyols)
- asparagus (fructans, fructose, and polyols)

There are also foods that have both fructans and galactans, like some pulses and nuts. Since polyols (especially sorbitol) are the FODMAPs most likely to be found with other FODMAPs, I'll explain how to reintroduce them. You have two options when dealing with foods that contain polyols in addition to another FODMAP:

1. Challenge the polyol group first. If you have a reaction to foods containing only polyols, then you know it's very likely you'll have a reaction to foods containing two FODMAPs, because most of those foods contain polyols.

OR

2. Choose any group, without testing the polyols first, and leave the foods that contain polyols for the last challenge.

Reintroduction, Group by Group

Which foods you decide to reintroduce within each category is up to you. I based my selection on foods I would be the most excited to bring back into my diet. Think of what foods you miss the most or what foods would make the diet easier or less stressful for you to follow.

Below are examples of foods you can test in each group. The serving sizes provided are to give you some guidance; you can try larger quantities on the days you're trying to push your limits or take several days and increase portions slowly. Remember that you can pick the foods you miss the most; you don't need to use the particular foods I'm providing below as an example. This is about finding what works for you.

Note: After each challenge group, it's important to go back to your elimination diet for five to seven days, even if you didn't have symptoms. Doing so prepares you for your next challenge. So after you challenge lactose, return to the elimination diet before challenging polyols or another group.

LACTOSE

DAY 1 (CAUTIOUS CHALLENGE): 3 ounces Greek yogurt
DAY 2 (MODERATE AMOUNT): 6 ounces (1 container) Greek yogurt
DAY 3 (PUSH YOUR LIMITS): 8 ounces milk with breakfast; 2 tablespoons cream cheese with a gluten-free bagel; ½ cup ice cream with dinner

POLYOLS

DAY 1 (CAUTIOUS CHALLENGE): ¼ cup avocado

DAY 2 (MODERATE AMOUNT): ½ cup blackberries

DAY 3 (PUSH YOUR LIMITS): sugar-free gum containing sorbitol *or* include ½ cup avocado with lunch and ½ cup cauliflower with dinner

FRUCTOSE

DAY 1 (CAUTIOUS CHALLENGE): 3 spears asparagus or ½ cup mango

DAY 2 (MODERATE AMOUNT): 1 to 2 tablespoons honey with tea and 4 spears asparagus

DAY 3 (PUSH YOUR LIMITS): granola that contains honey, dried fruit, and fructose for breakfast or snack; beverage with agave syrup

DAY 4* (COMBINE W/ POLYOLS): 1 medium apple or pear

*Note: Skip day 4 or be very careful if you've had a reaction to polyols or haven't tried them yet.

FRUCTANS

DAY 1 (CAUTIOUS CHALLENGE): 1 clove garlic or garlic powder

DAY 2 (MODERATE AMOUNT): cook your veggies with onions for lunch; prepare dinner with broth containing garlic and onions

DAY 3 (PUSH YOUR LIMITS): 1 to 2 slices wheat bread with breakfast; soup with garlic and onions for lunch; couscous with dinner

DAY 4* (COMBINE W/ POLYOLS): 7 to 10 pods snow peas or 1 cup mushrooms

*Note: Skip day 4 or be very careful if you've had a reaction to polyols or haven't tried them yet.

GALACTANS

DAY 1 (CAUTIOUS CHALLENGE): ⅛ cup cashews

DAY 2 (MODERATE AMOUNT): 2 tablespoons hummus with raw veggies for snack; ½ cup soaked lentils

DAY 3 (PUSH YOUR LIMITS): ½ cup beans

DAY 4* (COMBINE W/ POLYOLS): 1 cob sweet corn

*Note: Skip day 4 or be very careful if you've had a reaction to polyols or haven't tried them yet.

FODMAP REINTRODUCTION TRACKER

Use this table to track symptoms as you reintroduce foods from each FODMAP group. You can also download this form from callistomediabooks.com/lowfodmapforbeginners. Make as many copies as you need so you can continue to track symptoms as you reintroduce foods.

DATE	GROUP + FOOD	AMOUNT	SYMPTOMS
			☐ OKAY ☐ LIMIT ☐ AVOID
			☐ OKAY ☐ LIMIT ☐ AVOID
			☐ OKAY ☐ LIMIT ☐ AVOID
			☐ OKAY ☐ LIMIT ☐ AVOID
			☐ OKAY ☐ LIMIT ☐ AVOID
			☐ OKAY ☐ LIMIT ☐ AVOID
			☐ OKAY ☐ LIMIT ☐ AVOID
			☐ OKAY ☐ LIMIT ☐ AVOID
			☐ OKAY ☐ LIMIT ☐ AVOID
			☐ OKAY ☐ LIMIT ☐ AVOID
			☐ OKAY ☐ LIMIT ☐ AVOID

Low-FODMAP Long Term

There has not been substantial research done looking at the long-term effects of following a low-FODMAP diet, as opposed to discontinuing it after six to eight weeks. For some people, staying on the low-FODMAP diet is the only way to find relief. Long term, you may need to supplement with certain minerals and vitamins to compensate for missing nutrients, which is something to discuss with your doctor and/or dietitian. Vitamin D, B vitamins, iron, and calcium are examples of nutrients that may need to be supplemented. There is a "modified low-FODMAP diet," which mostly focuses on a low-FODMAP diet with a few high-FODMAP foods that a person can tolerate. This is a less restrictive approach and does not necessarily require a two-step process. However, this has not been proven to be an effective method or to have the same results as going through the elimination and then reintroduction phases.

ALCOHOL AND FODMAPS

Certain types of alcohol are allowed with a low-FODMAP diet, but since alcohol is an irritant to the gut, it's recommended to limit your intake to one glass per day and preferably not every day. Alcohol is a common trigger for people who suffer from IBS. Alcohols like beer, vodka, whiskey, and gin are safe with the low-FODMAP diet (but keep in mind that beer is not gluten-free, so if you have celiac disease or are gluten intolerant, you should look for a gluten-free beer). Some wines, like dessert wines, are high in FODMAPs, as is rum. Stay away from most drink mixers except club soda, as they can have hidden FODMAP triggers like high-fructose corn syrup and agave syrup. Be careful of juice concentrates, too, since these can be high in FODMAPs as well.

Listening to Your Body

One of the most important lessons I've learned on this diet is to follow your gut—literally. Once you've completed the reintroduction process, you'll have a better understanding of what foods to avoid going forward. Of course, you can always "cheat," but it's important to know the results and implications of eating a food that makes you feel sick. For me, having a "cheat" snack or meal is not worth the resulting digestive discomfort, but for others it's well worth it.

This doesn't mean that if you follow the diet strictly, your old, familiar symptoms will never resurface. They can pop up due to difficult circumstances or life stressors; after all, there's a strong connection between the brain and the gut. If this does happen, reset your stomach by doing the elimination diet for a week. It's reassuring for both the mind and body to know you have some level of control over your symptoms and that there's something you can do to feel better. Also, be sure to address your stress levels and find ways to cope, like yoga, exercise, coloring, or meditation.

PART 2

Low-FODMAP Recipes

The recipes in this book are all low-FODMAP and gluten-free, and most contain no more than five ingredients (not counting oils, salt, and pepper). Where applicable, you'll see one or more of these dietary labels for dairy-free, vegetarian, or vegan recipes: **DAIRY FREE** **VEG** **VEGAN**

Here are a few other labels you'll see, and what they mean:

QUICK PREP All prep work can be done in 10 minutes or less

30 MIN The entire recipe takes 30 mins or less, start to finish

ONE POT The recipe can be made in a single cooking vessel

Additionally, the recipes include helpful tips to enhance your cooking experience and FODMAP knowledge. These tips run the gamut from substitution tips or allergen tips to prep or make-ahead suggestions.

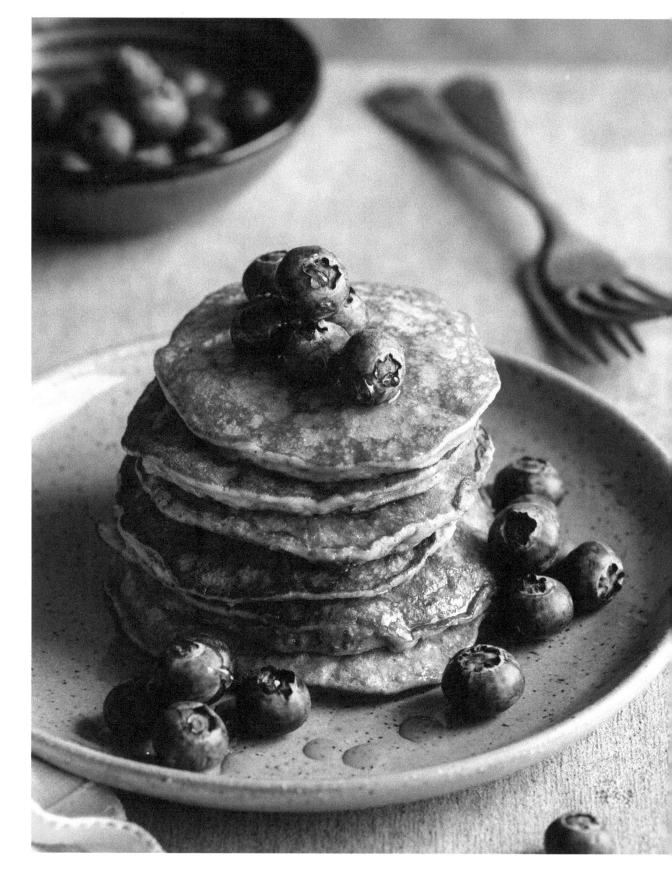

Chapter 5

Breakfast, Smoothies, and Drinks

Left: Banana Pancakes

BANANA PANCAKES

Serves 2

PREP TIME: 5 MINUTES / COOK TIME: 6 MINUTES

I grew up on the "funny face" pancake from a popular American diner that my parents would let me order on special occasions. And to this day, pancakes are one of my favorite breakfasts to make on a lazy weekend. These are an almost completely flour-free version yet are still light and fluffy like a traditional pancake. They're healthier, too, so there's no guilt in having a second serving! Feel free to top the pancakes with a handful of blueberries (no more than ½ cup) before diving in.

2 eggs

1 banana, mashed

1 tablespoon chia seeds

1 tablespoon brown rice flour

1 teaspoon vanilla extract

1 teaspoon cinnamon

Nonstick cooking spray

SUBSTITUTION TIP: To make these pancakes vegan, omit the eggs from the recipe. Mix the chia seeds with 2 tablespoons of hot water and let them stand for 5 minutes, until all the water is absorbed. Give the seeds a stir, then prepare the pancake batter starting with step 2. The texture and consistency of the pancakes will change very little from those made with eggs.

1. Whisk the eggs in a medium bowl.

2. Add the banana, chia seeds, brown rice flour, vanilla, and cinnamon to the bowl, and mix until well combined.

3. Heat a large skillet or griddle over medium-high heat. Spray the bottom of the skillet with the cooking spray.

4. Pour 2 heaping tablespoonfuls of batter per pancake onto the skillet and cook for 1 to 2 minutes, or until bubbles begin to form on the top of each pancake and the bottom is golden brown. Flip the pancakes and cook until the bottoms are golden brown, 1 to 2 minutes.

PER SERVING (3 pancakes) Calories: 168; Carbohydrates: 19g; Fat: 8g; Protein: 9g; Fiber: 5g; Sodium: 186mg

EASY FRENCH TOAST

Serves 2

PREP TIME: 5 MINUTES / COOK TIME: 6 MINUTES

French toast is an American breakfast staple traditionally made with dense bread dipped in an egg wash. This recipe boosts the traditional flavor profile with vanilla and cinnamon. Feel free to let your creativity run wild by adding different flavors like orange zest and nutmeg to your mix. I recommend Udi's gluten-free white bread because not only is it gluten-free, it's also free of high-FODMAP ingredients such as high-fructose corn syrup, honey, and inulin. To make this recipe vegan, follow the substitution tip I include with Banana Pancakes on the previous page.

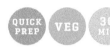

2 egg whites

1 tablespoon lactose-free milk, or almond or rice milk

1 teaspoon vanilla extract

1 teaspoon ground cinnamon

Nonstick cooking spray

4 slices gluten-free bread

SERVING TIP: For a little extra low-FODMAP sweetness, serve each portion with 1 tablespoon of maple syrup and ½ cup of sliced bananas and strawberries.

INGREDIENT TIP: I love incorporating cinnamon into this egg wash not only for the delicious flavor it adds but also for the multitude of health benefits. Cinnamon is full of healthy antioxidants, has anti-inflammatory properties, and protects against heart disease.

1. In a medium bowl, whisk together the egg whites, milk, vanilla, and cinnamon.

2. Heat a large skillet or griddle over medium-low heat. Once hot, spray the skillet with the cooking spray.

3. Working in batches if needed, dip each slice of bread into the wet mix until well coated on both sides. Add the slices to the skillet and cook for 3 minutes on each side, or until golden brown.

PER SERVING (2 pieces) Calories: 272; Carbohydrates: 42g; Fat: 9g; Protein: 8g; Fiber: 3g; Sodium: 657mg

VEGETABLE FRITTATA

Serves 4

PREP TIME: 5 MINUTES / COOK TIME: 25 MINUTES

I love being able to make a dish that has more than one use. This frittata is great for lunch and dinner, too, whether it's made specifically for those meals or served as leftovers. Frittatas are also a great way to include both vegetables and protein in your meal.

6 eggs

1 medium tomato, diced

½ cup black olives

¼ cup chopped scallions

½ cup shredded mozzarella cheese

Pinch sea salt

Freshly ground black pepper

1. Preheat the oven to 400°F.

2. Whisk the eggs and a splash of water in a large bowl. Set aside.

3. Distribute the tomato, olives, scallions, and cheese across a 9-by-9-inch baking dish or cast iron skillet. Pour the eggs into the dish, and season with salt and pepper.

4. Bake for 20 to 25 minutes, or until the eggs are set. Let the frittata cool for 5 minutes before slicing it.

SUBSTITUTION TIP: To include proteins like sausage or bacon in the frittata, add them in step 3 before pouring the eggs into the dish.

PER SERVING (2 pieces) Calories: 144; Carbohydrates: 4g; Fat: 10g; Protein: 11g; Fiber: 1g; Sodium: 315mg

BREAKFAST QUINOA

Makes 3½ cups

PREP TIME: 5 MINUTES / COOK TIME: 20 MINUTES

My husband pokes fun at my obsession with quinoa, but who can blame me with all the amazing health benefits packed into this little grain? This breakfast dish is a pleasant alternative to oatmeal that still ticks off all the boxes for a warm and satisfying breakfast. Even better, it can be made on a Sunday and enjoyed throughout the week. Just heat it up in the microwave before serving.

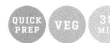

½ cup unsweetened coconut shreds

2 cups nondairy milk of your choice

1 cup uncooked quinoa

¼ cup maple syrup

1 tablespoon chia seeds

1. In a medium saucepan over medium heat, lightly toast the coconut shreds, stirring occasionally so they don't burn. Transfer the coconut to a bowl, and set aside to cool.

2. In the same saucepan, bring the milk, quinoa, maple syrup, and chia seeds to a boil. Reduce the heat to low, cover the pan, and cook until the quinoa is tender and the liquid is absorbed, 15 to 20 minutes.

INGREDIENT TIP: Feel free to add your favorite flavorings, like cinnamon or fresh berries, while the quinoa cooks. It's a great dish to experiment with.

PER SERVING (about 1¼ cups) Calories: 618; Carbohydrates: 74g; Fat: 30g; Protein: 14g; Fiber: 12g; Sodium: 120mg

BAKED VEGETABLE EGG MUFFINS

Makes 10 muffins

PREP TIME: 10 MINUTES / COOK TIME: 20 MINUTES

I make these egg muffins almost every Sunday to have throughout the entire week. The eggs are already portioned out, which makes for a perfect grab-and-go breakfast. And there are so many substitutions and variations you can make that your egg muffins will never become boring.

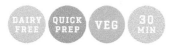

Nonstick cooking spray

½ cup diced green bell pepper

½ cup chopped spinach

5 eggs

5 egg whites

1 medium tomato, diced

Pinch sea salt

Freshly ground black pepper

1. Preheat the oven to 350°F. Spray the cups of a muffin tin with the cooking spray.

2. Heat a nonstick skillet over medium heat. Add the bell pepper and sauté it for 3 minutes. Add the spinach to the pan and continue sautéing for 2 minutes more.

3. Whisk both the whole eggs and egg whites in a large bowl. Add the sautéed vegetables and the tomato, and season with salt and pepper. Stir to combine.

4. Fill each of 10 muffin cups three-quarters full with the egg mixture. Bake for 18 to 20 minutes, or until the eggs are set.

MAKE-AHEAD TIP: These egg muffins can easily be kept frozen. Just transfer the cooled muffins into individual zip-top plastic bags and freeze them for up to 1 month. When you're ready to eat them, reheat them in the oven or microwave.

PER SERVING (2 muffins) Calories: 98; Carbohydrates: 2g; Fat: 5g; Protein: 10g; Fiber: 1g; Sodium: 132mg

BAKED BLUEBERRY OATMEAL CUPS

Makes 12 oatmeal cups

PREP TIME: 5 MINUTES / COOK TIME: 20 MINUTES

My mom enjoys instant oatmeal with fresh blueberries every single morning, and even brings it on the road with her when she goes out of town. This is my take on her daily bowl of oatmeal and blueberries. One batch of these oatmeal cups will last you the entire week. Reheat them for 20 seconds in the microwave, and you're ready to get your morning started.

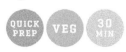

2 cups rolled oats (choose gluten-free if needed)

¼ teaspoon sea salt

1 egg

¾ cup lactose-free milk of your choice

¼ cup maple syrup

¾ cup blueberries

SUBSTITUTION TIP: Experiment with other low-FODMAP fruits like strawberries or raspberries in place of blueberries. I love to buy berries in bulk in the summer and freeze them to use when they're out of season.

MAKE-AHEAD TIP: These oatmeal cups freeze well. Place each serving in a zip-top plastic bag and freeze for up to 1 month.

1. Preheat the oven to 350°F. Line 12 muffin cups with paper liners.

2. In a medium bowl, combine the oats and salt. Set aside.

3. In a large bowl, whisk together the egg, milk, and maple syrup. Add the oats to the bowl, and mix until well combined. Gently fold in the blueberries.

4. Fill each muffin cup three-quarters full.

5. Bake for 18 to 20 minutes, or until the oatmeal has set and the tops are lightly browned.

PER SERVING (2 oatmeal cups) Calories: 120; Carbohydrates: 22g; Fat: 2g; Protein: 4g; Fiber: 2g; Sodium: 105mg

SALTY & SWEET GRANOLA

Makes 4 cups

PREP TIME: 10 MINUTES / COOK TIME: 30 MINUTES

Granola is one of my favorite go-to breakfast staples and makes for a perfect snack as well. I eat mine with nondairy milk or lactose-free yogurt. Most store-bought versions are full of sugar and processed ingredients, but this homemade version is FODMAP safe. The best part is, it will stay fresh in the pantry as long as you keep it in an airtight container.

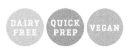

¼ cup coconut oil

2 cups old-fashioned oats

½ cup sunflower seeds

¼ cup maple syrup

¼ cup walnuts or pecans

¼ teaspoon sea salt

1. Preheat the oven to 325°F. Line a baking sheet with parchment paper.

2. In a large microwave-safe bowl, melt the coconut oil in the microwave.

3. To the bowl, add the oats, sunflower seeds, maple syrup, walnuts, and salt. Mix until well combined.

4. Spread the oats in a thin, even layer on the baking sheet.

5. Bake for 25 to 30 minutes, stirring once, until golden brown.

ALLERGEN TIP: If you're nut-free, swap out the walnuts or pecans with another seed like pumpkin seeds, or double the amount of sunflower seeds in the recipe.

PER SERVING (½ cup) Calories: 271; Carbohydrates: 18g; Fat: 21g; Protein: 4g; Fiber: 4g; Sodium: 66mg

CHOCOLATE CHIA PUDDING

Makes 1 cup

PREP TIME: 5 MINUTES, PLUS OVERNIGHT TO CHILL

I have a major sweet tooth, and this pudding satisfies my cravings. Chia seeds have so many wonderful health benefits, such as being high in omega-3 fatty acids, fiber, and antioxidants. The chia seeds expand overnight to create a thick pudding-like texture. Plus it can be eaten for breakfast too! To keep this recipe low-FODMAP, the portion size is pretty small, so for a more complete breakfast pair this with a couple of scrambled eggs.

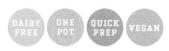

1¼ cups full-fat canned coconut milk

¼ cup chia seeds

3 tablespoons high-quality cocoa powder

2 tablespoons maple syrup

¼ teaspoon sea salt

1. In a glass jar with a resealable lid, combine the coconut milk, chia seeds, cocoa powder, maple syrup, and salt. Tightly seal the jar and shake it until the ingredients are well combined.

2. Refrigerate overnight, and serve chilled.

SUBSTITUTION TIP: This is a basic chia pudding recipe that you can expand on by adding vanilla extract, cinnamon, and fresh mint. The options are endless. Experiment with different flavors to find those that satisfy your sweet tooth.

INGREDIENT TIP: Unused canned coconut milk can be used to make Thai Coconut Cod (page 89).

PER SERVING (⅓ cup) Calories: 357; Carbohydrates: 24g; Fat: 31g; Protein: 7g; Fiber: 11g; Sodium: 173mg

GREEN MONSTER SMOOTHIE

Makes 2 servings

PREP TIME: 2 MINUTES

I love making smoothies that are packed with healthy doses of fruit and vegetables. Don't let the bright-green color fool you: You can't even taste the spinach, but you still get all its nutrients. This recipe serves two, but you can always freeze the second portion for another time. Simply thaw and blend it up when you're ready for it.

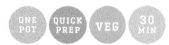

2 cups lactose-free milk, or almond or rice milk

1 medium banana (unripe)

1 cup fresh or frozen spinach

½ cup frozen pineapple chunks

Place the milk, banana, spinach, and pineapple chunks in a blender, and blend until smooth.

———————

PER SERVING (1 cup) Calories: 198; Carbohydrates: 31g; Fat: 5g; Protein: 9g; Fiber: 2g; Sodium: 128mg

STRAWBERRY SPLIT SMOOTHIE

Makes 2 servings

PREP TIME: 2 MINUTES

This is my grown-up smoothie version of an ice cream banana split. I've found not using a straw to drink really helps reduce excess bloating and gas—oh, and not drinking the smoothie in under 2 minutes (like I tend to do) helps as well. Keep in mind that this recipe really makes two servings, so don't drink it all in one sitting (even if slowly), or those symptoms you're trying to avoid may come right back.

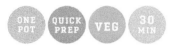

1 frozen banana (unripe)

2 cups lactose-free or nondairy milk

1 cup strawberries (about 10 medium-size)

2 tablespoons chia seeds

Place the banana, milk, strawberries, and chia seeds in a blender, and blend until smooth.

SUBSTITUTION TIP: Feel free to omit the chia seeds if you can't find them or haven't had a chance to restock your pantry. You can swap the chia for the same amount of ground flaxseeds for more protein, or add ¼ cup of old-fashioned, gluten-free oats to make the smoothie more filling.

PER SERVING (1 cup) Calories: 261; Carbohydrates: 37g; Fat: 10g; Protein: 12g; Fiber: 8g; Sodium: 116mg

LEMON-CUCUMBER COOLER

Makes about 1 gallon

PREP TIME: 2 MINUTES

When you're following the low-FODMAP diet, it can be hard to find safe beverages to drink. This super-refreshing drink is made with only tonic water, lemon, and cucumber. This is a major thirst quencher and will leave you feeling like you just left the spa. Just make sure you get tonic water sweetened with cane sugar, not high-fructose corn syrup.

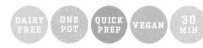

1 gallon tonic water

½ cucumber, thinly sliced

1 lemon, thinly sliced

Ice cubes

In a large pitcher, stir together the tonic water, cucumber, lemon, and ice cubes.

INGREDIENT TIP: I love adding fresh mint to my water to give it a pop of flavor.

PER SERVING (1 cup serving) Calories: 83; Carbohydrates: 23g; Fat: 0g; Protein: 0g; Fiber: 0g; Sodium: 18mg

GOLDEN MILK

Serves 4

PREP TIME: 2 MINUTES / COOK TIME: 2 MINUTES

Golden milk is the perfect comfort drink to have as a nightcap before going to bed. The ingredients remind me of a very simple take on chai. Turmeric has enormous benefits in the antioxidant, anti-inflammatory, and anti-cancer categories, and this drink is a great way to enjoy all those benefits. The pinch of ground pepper helps your body absorb the turmeric.

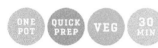

2 cups lactose-free or nondairy milk

1 tablespoon maple syrup

1 teaspoon cinnamon

1 teaspoon turmeric

Pinch freshly ground black pepper

1. In a small saucepan, bring the milk to a boil, then stir in the maple syrup, cinnamon, turmeric, and pepper.

2. Lower the heat to a simmer, cover the pan, and simmer for 10 minutes.

INGREDIENT TIP: If the drink isn't sweet enough for your taste, you can add an extra ½ tablespoon of maple syrup, as a 1½-tablespoon serving size is permitted on a low-FODMAP elimination diet. Be aware that only 100 percent maple syrup is cleared for use.

MAKE-AHEAD TIP: If you make this milk ahead of time or have leftovers, store it in an airtight container in the refrigerator for up to 1 week.

PER SERVING (½ cup) Calories: 78; Carbohydrates: 10g; Fat: 3g; Protein: 4g; Fiber: 0g; Sodium: 58mg

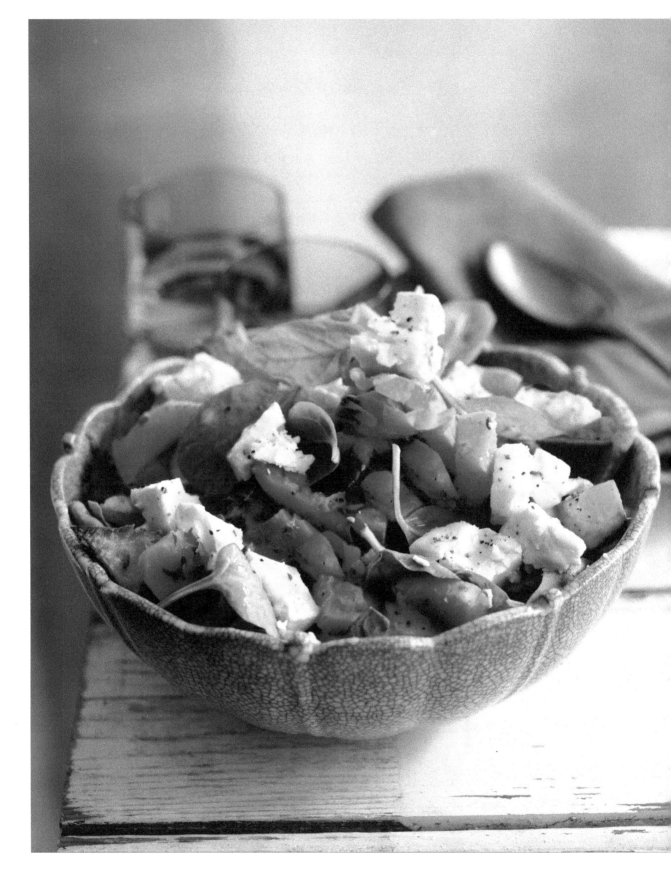

Vegetables and Salads

Left: Spinach Salad with Feta and Pumpkin Seeds

MISO EGGPLANT

Serves 4

PREP TIME: 10 MINUTES / COOK TIME: 30 MINUTES

I used to think I hated eggplant, but it turns out, I love it. I just didn't know how to properly prepare it. When made correctly, eggplant has a wonderful soft texture and absorbs so many flavors of the other ingredients it's prepared with. This miso eggplant is a fantastic side dish with the Vegetable Fried Rice (page 82) or Thai Coconut Cod (page 89).

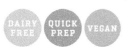

2 tablespoons miso paste

1 tablespoon mirin

1 tablespoon water

1 tablespoon sesame seeds

1 tablespoon minced fresh ginger (optional)

1 large eggplant

Nonstick cooking spray

INGREDIENT TIP: Miso paste is a traditional Japanese ingredient made from fermented soybeans. A little goes a long way.

1. Preheat the oven to 400°F. Line a baking sheet with parchment paper.

2. In a small bowl, whisk together the miso paste, mirin, water, sesame seeds, and ginger (if using). Set aside.

3. Cut off and discard the ends of the eggplant, then slice the eggplant in half lengthwise. Gently cut crisscross lines into the flesh of each eggplant half, making sure not to cut through the skin.

4. Spray a large skillet with the cooking spray and place it over medium-high heat. Once hot, place the eggplant halves cut-side down in the skillet and sear them for 4 to 5 minutes, until browned and slightly tender.

5. Transfer the eggplant cut-side up to the baking sheet. Brush the miso dressing over the top of the eggplant.

6. Bake for 20 to 25 minutes, or until the eggplant is tender when a fork is inserted.

PER SERVING (1 cup) Calories: 82; Carbohydrates: 14g; Fat: 2g; Protein: 5g; Fiber: 3g; Sodium: 351mg

GRILLED BOK CHOY

Serves 4

PREP TIME: 2 MINUTES / COOK TIME: 5 MINUTES

Bok choy is a type of Chinese cabbage used in many dishes, including chicken with veg-etables or my Thai Coconut Cod (page 89). What I love the most about this leafy green is that it's high in calcium, dietary fiber, vitamins, and minerals, and can be low-FODMAP in the right portions. It's a win-win across the board.

1 tablespoon sesame oil

4 whole bok choy

1 teaspoon sesame seeds

1. Heat the oil on a grill pan over medium-high heat.

2. Place the bok choy on the pan and grill each side for 2 to 3 minutes, or until grill marks form.

3. Remove the bok choy from the heat and sprinkle them with the sesame seeds.

INGREDIENT TIP: Soy sauce can be drizzled on the bok choy for additional flavor.

PER SERVING (1 cup) Calories: 134; Carbohydrates: 18g; Fat: 6g; Protein: 12g; Fiber: 8g; Sodium: 540mg

GRILLED PEPPERS, ZUCCHINI, AND CARROTS

Serves 4

PREP TIME: 10 MINUTES / COOK TIME: 20 MINUTES

I love anything cooked on the grill because of the natural flavors that come out. These vegetables are no exception. Grilled vegetables will turn the pickiest of kids and adults into vegetable lovers. The peppers, zucchini, and carrots in this recipe go well with my Greek Chicken Kebabs (page 100) and Dad's Easy Grilled Chicken (page 105).

1 (1-pound) bag mini yellow, red, and orange bell peppers

2 zucchini, cut into thick rounds

6 carrots, cut into thick rounds

2 tablespoons extra-virgin olive oil

1 teaspoon sea salt

Freshly ground black pepper

1. Heat an outdoor grill or grill pan to medium heat.

2. In a large bowl, add the bell peppers, zucchini, and carrots. Drizzle them with the olive oil, and season with salt and pepper. Toss to thoroughly coat the vegetables.

3. Grill the vegetables for 8 to 10 minutes on each side.

MAKE-AHEAD TIP: The vegetables can be grilled ahead of time and refrigerated in an airtight container for up to 1 week. They can be served reheated, cold, or at room temperature.

INGREDIENT TIP: Green bell peppers can contain high amounts of polyols (sorbitol) when served in amounts exceeding 1 cup. This recipe recommends a mix of red, orange, and yellow bell peppers to keep polyols in check.

PER SERVING (1 cup) Calories: 132; Carbohydrates: 17g; Fat: 7g; Protein: 3g; Fiber: 5g; Sodium: 571mg

SMASHED POTATOES

Serves 6

PREP TIME: 5 MINUTES / COOK TIME: 45 MINUTES

Smashed potatoes bring me back to eating drive-through tater tots as a kid. This recipe is just as addictive as those tots, but a lot healthier. The potatoes are great to make in large batches to be eaten throughout the week.

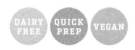

6 Yukon gold potatoes of uniform size

Extra-virgin olive oil

2 sprigs fresh rosemary, leaves removed and stems discarded

Sea salt

Freshly ground black pepper

1. Preheat the oven to 450°F. Line a baking sheet with parchment paper.

2. Bring a pot of salted water to a boil. Add the whole potatoes and cook until tender, about 25 minutes. Drain.

3. Transfer the potatoes to the baking sheet. Using a potato masher or the bottom of a cup, gently smash the potatoes. Drizzle each potato with olive oil, sprinkle with the rosemary leaves, and season with salt and pepper.

4. Bake for 20 minutes, or until the potatoes are golden brown on top.

INGREDIENT TIP: Try topping the potatoes with fresh or dried herbs like rosemary or paprika, or even low-FODMAP cheese (such as Cheddar, Colby, mozzarella, or Swiss) if eating vegan isn't a priority.

PER SERVING (1 potato) Calories: 182; Carbohydrates: 39g; Fat: 2g; Protein: 5g; Fiber: 3g; Sodium: 50mg

SESAME-SOY GREEN BEANS

Serves 6

PREP TIME: 5 MINUTES / COOK TIME: 7 MINUTES

I used to think all green beans tasted the way they do out of a can. But there's nothing tinny about fresh green beans! I can eat fresh green beans like French fries. I always order green beans when I go out for Chinese or Thai food. After I finally tried making them with soy and sesame at home, I realized I didn't need to go out to get my green-bean fix.

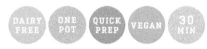

1 tablespoon sesame oil

1 pound green beans

2 teaspoons tamari or soy sauce

Pinch brown sugar

Heat the oil in a large skillet over medium-high heat. When the oil is hot, add the green beans, tamari, and sugar. Sauté for 5 to 7 minutes, or until the beans reach your desired tenderness.

ALLERGEN TIP: Soy sauce is permitted on the low-FODMAP diet, but it does contain wheat. If you have Celiac disease or gluten intolerance, choose gluten-free soy sauce or wheat-free tamari.

INGREDIENT TIP: Green beans can be high in polyols (sorbitol) if you eat more than about 17 of them. So while the portion size isn't terribly restrictive, it's good to keep in mind that green beans are not something you can eat without limit.

PER SERVING (1 cup) Calories: 44; Carbohydrates: 5g; Fat: 2g; Protein: 2g; Fiber: 3g; Sodium: 116mg

RATATOUILLE

Serves 4

PREP TIME: 10 MINUTES / COOK TIME: 30 MINUTES

This stew-like roasted-vegetable dish sounds way more gourmet than it actually is. It's rustic food at its best. I love surprising people by making something that's actually super easy but has a presentation that makes it appear very complicated. Another perk is that the flavors of the dish only get better a day or two later—that is, if you have any left over.

1 (14.5-ounce) can diced tomatoes

1 large eggplant, thinly sliced

1 yellow squash, thinly sliced

1 zucchini, thinly sliced

½ teaspoon sea salt

1 teaspoon dried oregano

1 teaspoon dried thyme

Extra-virgin olive oil or garlic-infused olive oil

1. Preheat the oven to 350°F.

2. In a small baking dish or cast iron skillet, spread the tomatoes and their juices across the bottom. Layer the eggplant, squash, and zucchini slices, alternating overlapping slices, on top of the tomatoes, working from the outer edge of the pan to the center in a spiral pattern.

3. Sprinkle the vegetables with the salt, oregano, and thyme, and drizzle with olive oil.

4. Bake for 30 minutes, or until the tomatoes are bubbling and the vegetables are tender.

MAKE-AHEAD TIP: This dish makes for great leftovers as the flavors get better and better. You can double the recipe to have vegetables for the week. Store in the refrigerator in an airtight container.

PER SERVING (1 cup) Calories: 77; Carbohydrates: 15g; Fat: 2g; Protein: 3g; Fiber: 7g; Sodium: 254mg

STUFFED TOMATOES WITH BREAD CRUMBS, SPINACH, AND MOZZARELLA

Serves 4

PREP TIME: 15 MINUTES / COOK TIME: 30 MINUTES

Stuffed tomatoes are easy to cook and also make for a great presentation. The addition of the mozzarella and bread crumbs makes this a satisfying side dish to almost any meal. There are many different variations of stuffed tomatoes that you can prepare; this happens to be one of my favorites.

1 teaspoon extra-virgin olive oil or garlic-infused olive oil

2 cups chopped spinach

Sea salt

1 cup gluten-free bread crumbs

1 tablespoon fresh parsley or 1 teaspoon dried parsley

Freshly ground black pepper

4 beefsteak tomatoes

½ cup shredded mozzarella

ALLERGEN TIP: If you follow a dairy-free or vegan diet, feel free to omit the cheese. The tomatoes are just as delicious without it.

PER SERVING (1 tomato) Calories: 72; Carbohydrates: 11g; Fat: 2g; Protein: 3g; Fiber: 3g; Sodium: 158mg

1. Preheat the oven to 375°F.

2. Heat the olive oil in a large skillet over medium heat. Add the chopped spinach, season it with salt, and sauté just until it begins to wilt, 3 to 4 minutes. Remove the skillet from the heat.

3. In a medium bowl, add the bread crumbs, parsley, and wilted spinach. Season with the black pepper. Set aside.

4. Cut the tops of the tomatoes off and gently scoop out the pulp and seeds from each tomato. Blot the inside of each tomato with a paper towel to remove any excess liquid. Generously salt the inside of the tomatoes.

5. Stuff the tomatoes with the bread-crumb mixture and place them in an 8-by-8-inch baking dish. Cover with aluminum foil, and bake for 20 minutes.

6. Add the cheese to the tops of the tomatoes, then re-cover and bake for 5 minutes more.

LEMON SAUTÉED SPINACH

Serves 8

PREP TIME: 5 MINUTES / COOK TIME: 5 MINUTES

I grew up thinking that in order to be big and strong like Popeye, you had to eat spinach. This recipe is in honor of all the other kids who were tricked into eating spinach. The fresh citrus flavor of this recipe really stands out and makes for a perfect side dish with the Chicken Piccata (page 102) or Baked Salmon (page 87).

1 teaspoon extra-virgin olive oil or garlic-infused olive oil

1 (1-pound) bag baby spinach

Pinch sea salt

Freshly squeezed lemon juice

1. Heat the olive oil in a large pan over medium heat. Add the spinach and salt. Sauté for 3 to 4 minutes, or until the spinach has wilted.

2. Remove the pan from the heat and stir a squeeze of lemon juice into the spinach.

INGREDIENT TIP: Using freshly squeezed lemon juice gives sometimes-bland spinach an extra boost of fresh, vibrant flavor.

PER SERVING (½ cup) Calories: 20; Carbohydrates: 2g; Fat: 1g; Protein: 2g; Fiber: 1g; Sodium: 82mg

THE BASIC SALAD

Serves 4

PREP TIME: 5 MINUTES / COOK TIME: 2 MINUTES

I love the basics when it comes to salad. It takes only a few quality ingredients to make this salad stand out. The ingredients may be simple, but the flavors and healthy nutrients are anything but.

¼ cup pumpkin seeds

1 (1-pound) bag arugula

½ cup cherry tomatoes

½ cucumber, thinly sliced

2 tablespoons Basic Vinaigrette (page 130)

1. In a medium skillet over medium heat, toast the pumpkin seeds for 1 to 2 minutes, stirring frequently so they don't burn. Remove the skillet from the heat.

2. In a serving bowl, add the arugula, pumpkin seeds, tomatoes, and cucumbers. Right before serving, drizzle with the salad dressing and toss to combine.

INGREDIENT TIP: If you decide not to make homemade dressing and opt for a store-bought version, be cautious. Many prepared dressings contain hidden FODMAP triggers like garlic, onions, or milk.

PER SERVING (2 cups) Calories: 137; Carbohydrates: 5g; Fat: 8g; Protein: 3g; Fiber: 1g; Sodium: 18mg

FALL HARVEST SALAD

Serves 4

PREP TIME: 10 MINUTES / COOK TIME: 40 MINUTES

I love bringing this dish to our family Thanksgiving meal to add some variety to the traditional Thanksgiving casseroles. Plus, serving a dish that is super bright and colorful is a nice change of pace from the mainly beige Thanksgiving dishes. If you're not a huge fan of quinoa, white or brown rice is a fine substitute.

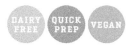

2 cups cubed acorn squash

1 teaspoon extra-virgin olive oil, plus
    additional to drizzle on the squash

Sea salt

Freshly ground black pepper

1 cup cooked Foolproof Quinoa (page 138)

1 cup arugula

½ cup toasted sunflower seeds

¼ cup pomegranate seeds

1. Preheat the oven to 400°F. Line a baking sheet with aluminum foil.

2. Add the squash to the baking sheet in a single layer, drizzle it with olive oil, and season with salt and pepper. Bake for 35 to 40 minutes, or until the squash is fork tender.

3. In a large bowl, combine the quinoa, roasted squash, arugula, sunflower seeds, pomegranate seeds, and 1 teaspoon of olive oil. Season with salt and pepper. Stir to combine.

PER SERVING (1 cup) Calories: 134; Carbohydrates: 18g; Fat: 6g; Protein: 4g; Fiber: 4g; Sodium: 28mg

TRADITIONAL GREEK SALAD

Serves 4

PREP TIME: 10 MINUTES

My husband and I went to Greece on our honeymoon, and I was enchanted with the beauty of the country. The fresh tomatoes and cucumbers, served with almost every meal, were out of this world. I was told the secret to the amazing flavors came from the saltwater breeze. I would happily eat this version of the salad for every meal, including breakfast.

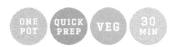

4 tomatoes, diced

1 cucumber, peeled and diced

¼ cup extra-virgin olive oil

¼ cup feta cheese or nondairy cheese

¼ teaspoon dried oregano

Kosher salt

In a large bowl, add the tomatoes, cucumber, olive oil, feta, oregano, and salt, and gently mix until well combined.

MAKE-AHEAD TIP: This salad can be made ahead of time, as the flavors become enhanced the longer the salad sits. Refrigerate in a resealable container for up to 1 week.

PER SERVING (1 cup) Calories: 166; Carbohydrates: 8g; Fat: 15g; Protein: 3g; Fiber: 2g; Sodium: 151mg

SPINACH SALAD WITH FETA AND PUMPKIN SEEDS

Serves 4

PREP TIME: 5 MINUTES

I always tell my family that their plate should be filled with color, not just beige foods. This salad is the most perfect example of a bowl of beautiful colors and flavors. It has even turned my usually salad-hating audience into true believers.

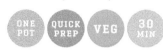

1 (1-pound) bag baby spinach

1 cup roasted butternut squash cubes

¼ cup pumpkin seeds

¼ cup feta cheese crumbles or nondairy cheese

Kosher salt

Extra-virgin olive oil

In a large bowl, add the spinach, squash, pumpkin seeds, and feta. Season with a sprinkle of salt, drizzle with olive oil, and gently mix until well combined.

MAKE-AHEAD TIP: To roast the squash, preheat the oven to 400°F. On a baking sheet lined with parchment paper, place the cubed squash in a single layer. Drizzle with olive oil and season with salt and pepper. Roast for 20 to 25 minutes, or until fork tender. If using for meals throughout the week, refrigerate in a resealable container.

PER SERVING (1 cup) Calories: 114; Carbohydrates: 9g; Fat: 7g; Protein: 7g; Fiber: 4g; Sodium: 224mg

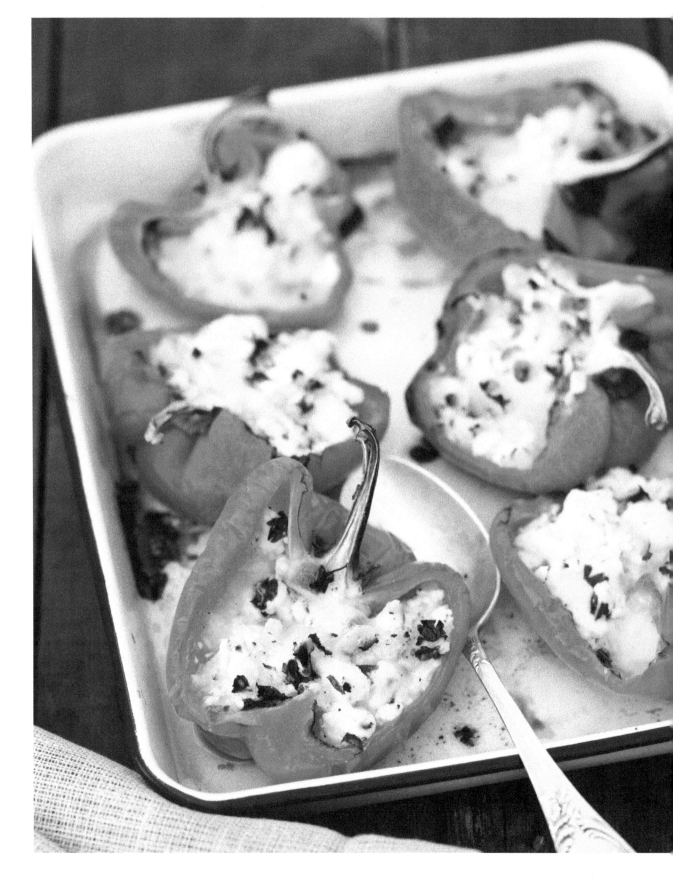

Meatless Mains

Left: Stuffed Red Peppers with Quinoa, Zucchini, and Feta Cheese

ZOODLES WITH TOMATO SAUCE

Serves 4

PREP TIME: 10 MINUTES / COOK TIME: 3 MINUTES

If you don't know what zoodles are, you're in for a treat. Zoodles are zucchini "noodles," created using a spiral slicer. Zoodles are a popular and delicious low-carb replacement for pasta. The first time I made zoodles for my husband, I was afraid he would revolt. I worry no more: He liked the crunch and texture of the "noodles." Plus everything tastes good with a fantastic sauce.

4 zucchini

1 teaspoon extra-virgin olive oil, plus
    additional if needed

Pinch sea salt

Freshly ground black pepper

1 cup Easy Pasta Sauce (page 137)

MAKE-AHEAD TIP: Zucchini can be made into "zoodles" ahead of time and kept in an airtight container in the refrigerator until ready to sauté. The key is to sauté them for only a minute, or you end up with soggy zoodles. I also like eating the zoodles raw topped with warm pasta sauce.

1. Cut off the ends of the zucchini, but do not peel the skin. If you have a spiral slicer, follow its instructions to make spaghetti-like zoodles. If you don't have a spiral slicer, a vegetable peeler can be used, too.

2. Heat the olive oil in a large skillet over medium-high heat. Add half the zoodles, and season with salt and pepper. Sauté the zoodles for about 1 minute, until slightly tender. Transfer these zoodles to a bowl and repeat with the remaining zoodles. If the pan seems dry, add a small drizzle more of olive oil.

3. In a small saucepan over medium heat, heat the pasta sauce. When hot, pour the sauce over the zoodles.

PER SERVING (1½ cups) Calories: 152; Carbohydrates: 13g; Fat: 11g; Protein: 4g; Fiber: 4g; Sodium: 100mg

STUFFED RED PEPPERS WITH QUINOA, ZUCCHINI, AND FETA CHEESE

Serves 4

PREP TIME: 10 MINUTES / COOK TIME: 30 MINUTES

I love being able to use leftovers from the week to make a completely new dish. These stuffed peppers in particular are a great way of using leftover grains and vegetables. If you've never had stuffed red peppers, you'll be delighted at how filling and satisfying they are.

1 teaspoon extra-virgin olive oil

1 zucchini, diced

2 cups Foolproof Quinoa (page 138)

Pinch sea salt

Freshly ground black pepper

4 bell peppers (red, orange, or yellow)

½ cup feta cheese crumbles (optional)

SUBSTITUTION TIP: This meatless dish can easily be made into a meat dish by stuffing the peppers with cooked ground meat.

1. Preheat the oven to 375°F.

2. Heat the olive oil in a medium skillet over medium-high heat. Add the zucchini and sauté until slightly tender, 2 to 3 minutes. Transfer the zucchini to a large bowl.

3. Add the quinoa to the bowl of zucchini, and season with salt and pepper. Stir to combine well. Set aside.

4. Cut off the tops of the bell peppers and remove the seeds and ribs from inside. Stuff the peppers with the quinoa mixture.

5. Place the stuffed peppers in an 8-by-8-inch baking dish. Cover with aluminum foil and bake for 20 minutes.

6. Remove the peppers from the oven and add the feta to the top of each pepper (if using). Re-cover with the foil and bake for an additional 5 minutes.

PER SERVING (1 pepper) Calories: 154; Carbohydrates: 27g; Fat: 3g; Protein: 6g; Fiber: 5g; Sodium: 90mg

CREAMY PUMPKIN PASTA

Serves 4

PREP TIME: 10 MINUTES / COOK TIME: 15 MINUTES

This dish reminds me of a decadent bowl of fettuccine Alfredo—but without the resulting FODMAP-related stomachache. The creaminess comes from the canned pumpkin and coconut milk. There are plenty of ways to get the palate–pleasing creaminess and texture of a dairy-free dish, and this is but one example. Though you'll be tempted to eat more, stick to only one serving of this dish at a time. In larger quantities, pumpkin purée and coconut milk may be high in FODMAPs.

1 (1-pound) package gluten-free pasta

1 cup pumpkin purée

½ cup light coconut milk

2 tablespoons water

Pinch sea salt

Freshly ground black pepper

1. Cook the pasta according to the package instructions.

2. While the pasta is cooking, in a large saucepan, whisk together the pumpkin purée and coconut milk, and bring to a boil.

3. Reduce the heat to low and let the sauce simmer for a few minutes. If the sauce is too thick, add some or all of the water to thin it out to your desired consistency. Season with salt and pepper.

4. Drain the pasta, immediately add it to the sauce, and stir to combine.

SUBSTITUTION TIP: If you're not a fan of coconut milk, you can use a lactose-free or nondairy milk instead.

PER SERVING (1 cup) Calories: 515; Carbohydrates: 90g; Fat: 10g; Protein: 16g; Fiber: 13g; Sodium: 46mg

ACORN SQUASH SOUP

Serves 6

PREP TIME: 10 MINUTES / COOK TIME: 2 HOURS

I love a big bowl of soup for lunch or dinner, but I've found it nearly impossible to order soup when dining out, due to the presence of FODMAP triggers like garlic and onion. This version is dairy-free, but even the toughest critic won't notice the lack of cream. I love making this soup and having it throughout the week.

Nonstick cooking spray

6 cups acorn squash, peeled and cubed

2 tablespoons extra-virgin olive oil

1 teaspoon sea salt, plus more for seasoning

2½ cups vegetable broth (without garlic, onion, or celery), divided

2 tablespoons chopped scallions

2 tablespoons unsalted butter (optional)

Freshly ground black pepper

PER SERVING (1 cup) Calories: 154; Carbohydrates: 26g; Fat: 5g; Protein: 1g; Fiber: 6g; Sodium: 2,085mg

1. Preheat the oven to 350°F. Line a large baking dish with aluminum foil and spray it with the cooking spray.

2. Add the squash, olive oil, and 1 teaspoon of salt to the baking dish, and stir to combine. Pour 1 cup of broth over the squash.

3. Bake for 90 minutes, stirring once after about 45 minutes so the squash doesn't stick to the foil. If there's no broth left in the dish, you can add a little more.

4. Transfer the squash and any leftover broth to a large Dutch oven pot. Turn the heat to medium-low and add the remaining 1½ cups of broth. Cook for 25 minutes.

5. Using an immersion blender, blend until the soup is completely smooth. Alternatively, add the soup to a blender, working in batches if necessary, and blend until smooth.

6. Stir in the scallions and butter (if using) until well combined. Season with pepper and additional salt if needed.

PASTA WITH FRESH BASIL, TOMATO, AND ZUCCHINI

Serves 4

PREP TIME: 10 MINUTES / COOK TIME: 12 MINUTES

This is my absolute favorite combination of pasta, vegetables, and fresh basil. It comes together quickly and makes for a perfect weeknight dinner. Fresh basil is my favorite herb to use in my cooking because it brings so much flavor to a dish. If you have fresh basil in your summer garden, I know you're always looking for ways to use its abundance. This is one of those ways.

1 (1-pound) package gluten-free pasta

1 teaspoon extra-virgin olive oil

1 cup cherry tomatoes

1 zucchini, diced

1 cup fresh basil

Pinch sea salt

Freshly ground black pepper

1. Cook the pasta according to the package instructions.

2. While the pasta cooks, heat the olive oil in a large pan over medium-high heat. Add the cherry tomatoes and zucchini, then sauté until the tomatoes burst, 6 to 8 minutes.

3. Top the pasta with the vegetables. Add the basil and stir to combine. Season with salt and pepper. Serve immediately.

INGREDIENT TIP: In my experience, I can never use a container of cherry or grape tomatoes fast enough before the tomatoes turn bad. Instead, I freeze them in a zip-top plastic bag and use them when needed.

PER SERVING (1 cup) Calories: 451; Carbohydrates: 86g; Fat: 4g; Protein: 15g; Fiber: 11g; Sodium: 46mg

SUMMER SPAGHETTI SQUASH

Serves 4

PREP TIME: 10 MINUTES / COOK TIME: 1 HOUR, 10 MINUTES

I got on the spaghetti squash bandwagon years ago when I realized it made for a perfect pasta substitute. I find that the easiest way to prepare the squash is to put the whole, uncut squash in the oven, instead of trying to cut it in half first. Trust me, it's considerably easier cutting the squash *after* it's been baked than before.

1 medium spaghetti squash
1 cup Sun-Dried Tomatoes (page 133)
1 cup chopped fresh spinach
½ cup roughly chopped fresh basil
1 tablespoon unsalted butter
1 tablespoon extra-virgin olive oil
Pinch sea salt
Freshly ground black pepper

INGREDIENT TIP: Spaghetti squash in amounts larger than 2½ cups can be high in fructans and galactans, so be mindful with how much you eat in one sitting.

MAKE-AHEAD TIP: This is a great dish to make ahead of time. Keep in an airtight container in the refrigerator for up to 5 days.

1. Preheat the oven to 375°F.

2. Using a fork, poke holes all over the squash. Place it in a baking dish and bake for 45 to 60 minutes, or until a fork is easily inserted.

3. Once the squash is cool enough to handle, cut it in half and carefully scrape out and discard the seeds, taking care not to scrape up the flesh.

4. Using a fork, scrape the squash into a large bowl. (The flesh will come out in spaghetti-like strings as it's scraped.)

5. Add the sun-dried tomatoes, spinach, basil, butter, and olive oil to the bowl. Season with salt and pepper, and stir until well combined.

PER SERVING (1 cup) Calories: 139; Carbohydrates: 18g; Fat: 8g; Protein: 3g; Fiber: 2g; Sodium: 353mg

VEGETABLE FRIED RICE

Serves 4

PREP TIME: 10 MINUTES / COOK TIME: 12 MINUTES

I love ordering fried rice when I'm out, but I have to specify no garlic and no onion, which is usually met with raised eyebrows. And no matter what, I finish my meal feeling heavy and overly full. I realized it was time to come up with my own version. This recipe is packed with vegetables and is much lighter than what you usually find in your local Chinese restaurant.

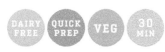

3 tablespoons sesame oil

¼ cup diced scallions

½ cup diced red bell pepper

½ cup shredded carrots

2 eggs

4 cups cooked brown rice

¼ cup tamari or soy sauce (gluten-free if necessary)

Juice of ½ lime

Fresh basil, for garnish (optional)

Fresh cilantro, for garnish (optional)

INGREDIENT TIP: Tofu, shrimp, or chicken can easily be added to this dish if you want a protein in there. Just cook the the protein in the pan and transfer it to a bowl before you cook the vegetables, then add it back to the pan when adding the rice and tamari.

1. In a large nonstick skillet or wok, heat the sesame oil over medium-high heat. Add the scallions and sauté for 1 to 2 minutes, or until softened.

2. Add the bell pepper and carrots, and sauté for 4 to 5 minutes, or until the vegetables just begin to get tender.

3. Move the vegetables around to the edge of the pan to leave the center clear. Crack the eggs into the middle of the pan. Begin to lightly scramble the eggs. Once the eggs are almost fully scrambled, mix them with the vegetables and continue stirring until the ingredients are well mixed and the eggs are fully cooked.

4. Add the cooked rice and tamari to the pan and mix well. Stir-fry until the rice begins to gently fry, 3 to 4 minutes.

5. Remove the pan from the heat and stir in the lime juice. Garnish with the basil and cilantro (if using).

PER SERVING (1 cup) Calories: 299; Carbohydrates: 36g; Fat: 14g; Protein: 8g; Fiber: 2g; Sodium: 1,052mg

TOFU AND BROWN RICE BOWL

Serves 4

PREP TIME: 30 MINUTES / COOK TIME: 45 MINUTES

What I love the most about cooking with tofu is that it takes on the flavor of the other ingredients in the dish. In this recipe, the most important thing to remember is to press the tofu for at least 20 to 30 minutes beforehand to remove the excess liquid.

1 (14-ounce) package firm tofu

2 cups brown rice

Pinch sea salt

Freshly ground black pepper

1 teaspoon sesame oil, plus additional to brown the tofu

2 cups fresh spinach

Juice of ½ lime

1 teaspoon minced fresh ginger (optional)

SUBSTITUTION TIP: The spinach can easily be swapped out for other vegetables like bok choy or eggplant. A combination of two or more vegetables is equally delicious.

PER SERVING (1 cup) Calories: 446; Carbohydrates: 76g; Fat: 8g; Protein: 17g; Fiber: 5g; Sodium: 92mg

1. Drain the tofu and place it on a paper-towel-lined plate. Put another paper towel on top of the tofu and weigh it down with another plate. Let stand for 30 minutes to remove the excess water. You will need to change the paper towels 2 to 3 times during this period.

2. Prepare the rice according to the package instructions.

3. While the rice cooks, cut the tofu into 2-inch rectangular pieces and season them with salt and pepper.

4. Heat a drizzle of sesame oil in a large pan over medium-high heat. Add the tofu and lightly brown it, 3 to 4 minutes per side. Transfer the tofu to a plate.

5. Heat 1 teaspoon of sesame oil in the pan over medium-high heat. Add the spinach and cook, stirring frequently, until it's wilted, 2 to 3 minutes.

6. Return the tofu to the pan and add the lime juice and ginger (if using). Stir to combine and serve with spinach over rice.

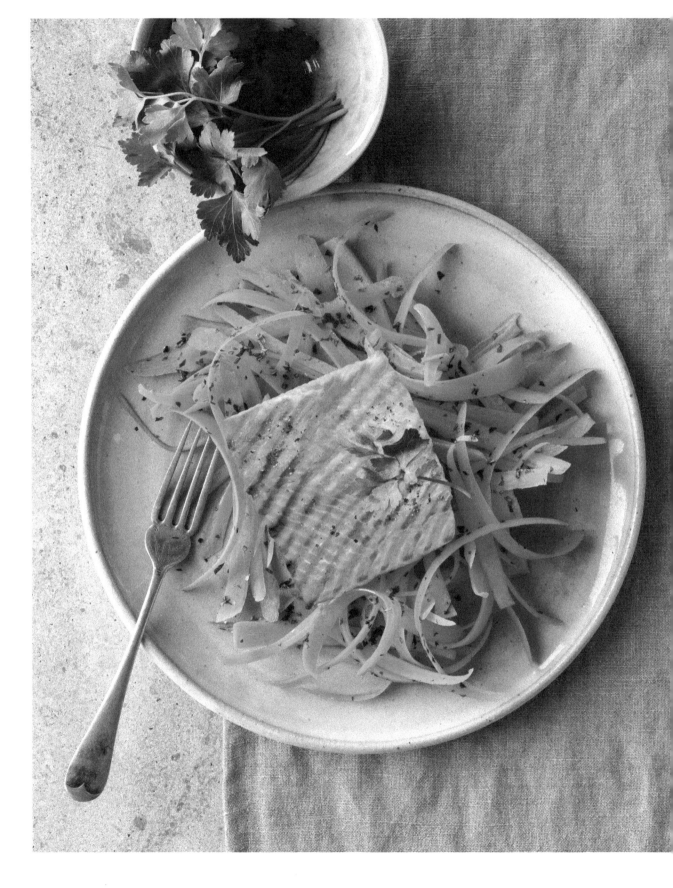

Chapter 8

Fish and Seafood

Left: Grilled Salmon with Carrot Ribbons

GRILLED SALMON WITH CARROT RIBBONS

Serves 2

PREP TIME: 10 MINUTES / COOK TIME: 10 MINUTES

If you ask me, there is an element about grilling that beats any other method of cooking. Not only is the cleanup a breeze, but the food tastes so much better with grill marks on it. I first learned this recipe after going to a friend's house for dinner and was blown away by how delicious the salmon turned out! Plus, who wants to worry about their kitchen smelling fishy after making dinner? Not me!

2 (6-ounce) salmon fillets

Sea salt

Freshly ground black pepper

1 pound whole carrots, skin peeled

Nonstick cooking spray

1 teaspoon extra-virgin olive oil, plus extra for the grill

1 tablespoon fresh parsley, loosely chopped

1. Preheat an outdoor grill on medium-high heat for 10 to 15 minutes.

2. Dry the fillets with paper towels, and season with salt and pepper.

3. Spray the cooking spray on the grill. Place each piece of salmon on it fillet-side down and skin-side up. Cook for 6 minutes, then flip and cook for an additional 4 minutes.

4. While the salmon cooks, use a vegetable peeler to peel the carrots into ribbons.

5. In a small bowl, toss the carrots with olive oil, and sprinkle with salt and the parsley. Serve the grilled salmon directly over the carrot ribbons.

PER SERVING Calories: 477; Carbohydrates: 23g; Fat: 22g; Protein: 38g; Fiber: 6g; Sodium: 392mg

BAKED SALMON

Serves 2

PREP TIME: 5 MINUTES / COOK TIME: 18 MINUTES

Salmon is one of the superfoods, and I try to incorporate it into my diet as much as I can. It has so many health benefits like combating heart disease, cancer, and cholesterol, to name just a few. The American Heart Association recommends consuming fatty fish like salmon at least twice a week. This recipe is an easy way to reach that twice-a-week goal, as it takes little time to cook.

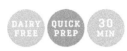

12 ounces salmon fillets

Sea salt

Freshly ground black pepper

1 tablespoon maple syrup

1 lemon, thinly sliced

1. Preheat the oven to 375°F. Line a baking sheet with parchment paper.

2. Place the salmon on the baking sheet and generously season it with salt and pepper. Drizzle the maple syrup over the salmon and layer the lemon slices atop the fish.

3. Bake for 15 to 18 minutes, or until cooked through.

SERVING TIP: This is a great dish to serve for a large dinner party, as there is little prep involved and the presentation is beautiful.

PER SERVING (6 ounces) Calories: 389; Carbohydrates: 7g; Fat: 20g; Protein: 36g; Fiber: 0g; Sodium: 165mg

PECAN-CRUSTED SALMON

Serves 2

PREP TIME: 5 MINUTES / COOK TIME: 18 MINUTES

I always want to order anything labeled "crusted" when I see it on a menu, but those items are almost always crusted with gluten- and FODMAP-laden bread crumbs. This recipe uses pecans instead of bread, which gives a great texture to the finished fish. Plus the flavor of the pecans, parsley, and mustard is out of this world.

Nonstick cooking spray

12 ounces salmon fillets

½ teaspoon sea salt

½ teaspoon freshly ground black pepper

1 tablespoon unsalted butter, melted

1 tablespoon Dijon mustard

2 teaspoons maple syrup

⅓ cup chopped pecans

1 tablespoon chopped fresh parsley

1. Preheat the oven to 400°F. Line a baking sheet with aluminum foil and spray it with the cooking spray.

2. Place the salmon fillets skin-side down on the baking sheet and season them with the salt and pepper.

3. In a small bowl, combine the melted butter, mustard, and maple syrup. Add the pecans and parsley to the bowl, and mix until well combined.

4. Pour the pecan mixture across the salmon, and use your fingers or the back of a spoon to lightly press it into the fish.

5. Bake for 15 to 18 minutes, or until the fish is cooked through and flakes easily.

ALLERGEN TIP: This dish is just as good without nuts—or you can substitute with pumpkin or sunflower seeds.

PER SERVING (6 ounces) Calories: 560; Carbohydrates: 7g; Fat: 38g; Protein: 39g; Fiber: 1g; Sodium: 142mg

THAI COCONUT COD

Serves 2

PREP TIME: 10 MINUTES / COOK TIME: 10 MINUTES

I came up with this recipe after always wanting to order a similar dish when eating out but not being able to because the restaurant-made sauce contains garlic and onion. I was determined to create my own version because I'm obsessed with anything made with coconut milk—it adds such a creamy texture to any dish. The best part is that this recipe is heavy on flavor but still tastes light and healthy. If you're not familiar with turmeric, it's a brightly colored anti-inflammatory spice that contains large quantities of antioxidants.

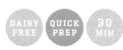

1 pound cod fillets

Pinch sea salt

Freshly ground black pepper

1½ teaspoons coconut oil

⅓ cup canned coconut milk

1 teaspoon curry powder

½ teaspoon ground turmeric

1 cup fresh spinach

Freshly squeezed lime juice (optional)

1. Season the cod on both sides with salt and pepper.

2. Heat the oil in a large skillet over medium heat. Add the cod to the pan and cook for 1 minute.

3. In a small bowl, whisk together the coconut milk, curry powder, and turmeric. Pour the mixture into the skillet with the fish, cover the pan, and cook for 5 minutes.

4. Turn the cod over, and add the spinach to the skillet. Cover the pan and cook for an additional 4 minutes, or until the fish is cooked through.

5. Remove the skillet from the heat and stir in a squeeze of lime juice (if using).

SUBSTITUTION TIP: Any firm white fish or shrimp works well in place of cod.

PER SERVING (½ fillet) Calories: 310; Carbohydrates: 4g; Fat: 12g; Protein: 41g; Fiber: 2g; Sodium: 256mg

PAN-FRIED COD

Serves 2

PREP TIME: 10 MINUTES / COOK TIME: 10 MINUTES

This recipe honors my love for fish and chips. On a visit to London, I let my fear of having a stomachache overtake my desire to try this traditional English dish, and missed my opportunity to try the "real deal." But I won't make that mistake twice. Until my next visit, this pan-fried cod will have to do. Luckily for me, it's pretty dang good.

1 cup rice flour

1 egg, lightly beaten

1 cup mashed-potato flakes

1 pound cod fillets

½ teaspoon sea salt

½ teaspoon freshly ground black pepper

2 tablespoons extra-virgin olive oil

1. Add the rice flour to a medium bowl, the beaten egg to another medium bowl, and the mashed-potato flakes to a third medium bowl.

2. One at a time, coat each cod fillet on both sides in the rice flour, then dip it completely in the egg, and finally coat it with the mashed-potato flakes. Season the fillets with the salt and pepper.

3. Heat the olive oil in a large skillet over medium-high heat. Pan-fry the fillets for about 4 minutes on each side, or until they're browned and flake easily with a fork.

INGREDIENT TIP: Mashed-potato flakes are from the boxes of instant mashed potatoes you find at the grocery store. They're my secret low-FODMAP, gluten-free ingredient for coating fish or chicken before baking or pan-frying.

PER SERVING (½ fillet) Calories: 493; Carbohydrates: 36g; Fat: 19g; Protein: 46g; Fiber: 3g; Sodium: 684mg

POACHED SNAPPER IN TOMATO-AND-BASIL SAUCE

Serves 2

PREP TIME: 5 MINUTES / COOK TIME: 13 MINUTES

In the summer, I want to spend less time in the kitchen and more time outside, which means putting together quick and easy dinner recipes. This healthy fish dish comes together super quickly and uses fresh summer flavors like basil and tomatoes. Serve the fish over a bowl of steamed rice or quinoa.

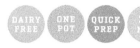

1 can diced tomatoes

¼ cup white wine

½ cup water

12 ounces red snapper fillets

1 teaspoon salt

Freshly ground black pepper

½ cup fresh basil leaves

1. In a medium pan over high heat, bring the tomatoes (including their juices), wine, and water to a boil.

2. While the tomatoes are coming to a boil, season both sides of the fish with salt and pepper.

3. Reduce the heat to medium and add the fish to the pan, making sure it's submerged in the liquid. Cover the pan and poach the fish for 8 to 10 minutes, or until it's cooked through.

4. Stir in the basil in the last minute of poaching the fish.

SUBSTITUTION TIP: If you're looking for a more affordable fish, a firm white fish like cod or tilapia is a perfect substitute for snapper.

PER SERVING (6 ounces) Calories: 276; Carbohydrates: 8g; Fat: 3g; Protein: 45g; Fiber: 2g; Sodium: 1,109mg

CORNMEAL-CRUSTED FISH
TACOS WITH COLESLAW

Serves 4

PREP TIME: 15 MINUTES / COOK TIME: 10 MINUTES

The way to my heart (and stomach) is through a good fish taco. This recipe does just that. The cornmeal crust gives the fish great texture and crunch without a greasy, heavy batter. Plus, cornmeal is naturally gluten-free and low-FODMAP, as it's made of ground, dried corn. The combination of the fish and coleslaw leads to the most perfect bite.

FOR THE FISH

½ cup cornmeal

1 tablespoon chili powder

½ teaspoon sea salt

4 tablespoons oil for frying (such as grapeseed, olive, or coconut oil), divided

2 pounds cod fillets, cut into 2-inch pieces

12 corn tortillas

FOR THE COLESLAW

4 cups cabbage, thinly sliced

2 tablespoons freshly squeezed lime juice

1 tablespoon extra-virgin olive oil

½ teaspoon apple cider vinegar

½ teaspoon maple syrup

Sea salt

Freshly ground black pepper

MAKE-AHEAD TIP: The coleslaw can be made in advance and refrigerated in an airtight container overnight.

PER SERVING (½ pound of fish) Calories: 565; Carbohydrates: 50g; Fat: 22g; Protein: 47g; Fiber: 8g; Sodium: 463mg

TO MAKE THE FISH

1. In a medium bowl, combine the cornmeal, chili powder, and salt. Set aside.

2. In a large skillet, heat 2 tablespoons of oil over medium-high heat.

3. Working in batches, coat the fish pieces with the cornmeal mixture. Gently shake off any excess cornmeal and add the fish to the skillet, making sure not to overcrowd the pieces.

4. Cook on each side until golden brown and cooked through, 2 to 3 minutes per side.

5. Transfer the fish to a paper-towel-lined baking sheet. Repeat steps 2 through 4 with the remaining fish.

TO MAKE THE COLESLAW

1. In a large bowl, combine the cabbage, lime juice, olive oil, vinegar, and maple syrup. Season with salt and pepper. Mix well and refrigerate until ready to serve.

2. Serve the fish, coleslaw, and tortillas, and let everyone build their own tacos.

BAKED COCONUT SHRIMP

Serves 4

PREP TIME: 10 MINUTES / COOK TIME: 10 MINUTES

I'm envious of my friends who get to order fried shrimp. I can never partake unless the menu specifies gluten-free. So instead of being jealous, I decided to make my own version, baked rather than fried, and coated in FODMAP-friendly coconut flakes and rice flour. They're so satisfying that no one will even know the difference. They're perfect as an appetizer or as a main dish along with a side of rice and vegetables.

2 eggs

1 cup dried unsweetened coconut flakes

2 tablespoons nutritional yeast

1 cup rice flour, divided

4 tablespoons cornstarch, divided

Sea salt

Freshly ground black pepper

16 large shrimp, peeled and deveined

1 tablespoon oil such as grapeseed oil, olive oil, or coconut oil

INGREDIENT TIP: Nutritional yeast is a deactivated yeast that has a nutty cheese-like flavor and is high in vitamin B. It's commonly used in a vegan diet as a replacement for the flavor of cheese.

1. Preheat the oven to 450°F. Line a baking sheet with parchment paper.

2. In a small bowl, whisk the eggs. Set aside.

3. In another small bowl, combine the coconut flakes, nutritional yeast, ½ cup of rice flour, 2 tablespoons of cornstarch, salt, and pepper. Set aside.

4. In a third small bowl, combine the remaining ½ cup of rice flour and 2 tablespoons of cornstarch.

5. One at a time, coat each shrimp in the flour-cornstarch mixture, dip it in the egg wash, then coat it in the coconut mixture. Place each shrimp on the baking sheet.

6. Drizzle the shrimp with the oil and bake for 5 minutes. Flip the shrimp over and bake for 4 to 5 minutes more, or until cooked through.

PER SERVING (4 shrimp) Calories: 296: Carbohydrates: 17g; Fat: 12g; Protein: 27g; Fiber: 2g; Sodium: 216mg

CRAB CAKES

Makes 4 crab cakes

PREP TIME: 20 MINUTES / COOK TIME: 8 MINUTES

Crab cakes are a staple in the Northeast, but that doesn't mean this Texas gal can't create her own version. These seem complicated to make but are actually quite easy to put together. (This is a meal that's ready in less than 30 minutes, after all.) The key is using high-quality ingredients, which allows the crab itself to stand out.

8 ounces lump crabmeat, drained

4 tablespoons gluten-free bread crumbs

1 tablespoon chopped scallions

1 tablespoon mayonnaise

1 teaspoon freshly grated lemon zest, plus more to garnish

1 egg, lightly beaten

Pinch sea salt

Freshly ground black pepper

1 tablespoon extra-virgin olive oil

1. In a medium bowl, gently combine the crab, bread crumbs, scallions, mayonnaise, lemon zest, and egg, and season with salt and pepper. Cover the bowl and chill the mixture in the refrigerator for at least 15 minutes to help bind the cakes.

2. Divide the crab mixture into 4 equal portions and shape them into 1-inch-thick patties.

3. Heat the olive oil in a large skillet over medium-high heat. Making sure the oil covers the bottom of the pan, carefully add the patties to the skillet and cook for 4 minutes on each side, or until the crab cakes are golden brown.

4. Transfer the crab cakes to a paper-towel-lined plate to drain any excess oil.

SERVING TIP: These crab cakes are delicious served over a bed of fresh arugula or spinach.

PER SERVING (1 cake) Calories: 261; Carbohydrates: 6g; Fat: 9g; Protein: 37g; Fiber: 0g; Sodium: 604mg

LEMONY PAN-SEARED SCALLOPS

Serves 4

PREP TIME: 5 MINUTES / COOK TIME: 6 MINUTES

Until recently, I had a fear of all things related to scallops, as I thought you had to be a real professional in the kitchen to cook them properly. How wrong I was! Turns out they're one of the easiest kinds of seafood to prepare. I'm so glad I faced my cooking fear and jumped on the scallop bandwagon.

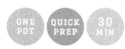

2 pounds sea scallops

Pinch sea salt

Freshly ground black pepper

2 tablespoons unsalted butter

Juice of ½ lemon

2 teaspoons chopped fresh parsley

1. Rinse the scallops and pat them dry with a paper towel. Season with salt and pepper.

2. Melt the butter in a large skillet over medium-high heat. Add the scallops to the pan, making sure not to crowd them together.

3. Let the scallops cook for 2 minutes without moving them, then turn over and let them cook for an additional 2 to 3 minutes, or until firm to the touch but still slightly soft.

4. Drizzle the scallops with the lemon juice and sprinkle with the parsley.

INGREDIENT TIP: Scallops are the perfect protein to serve over a salad, rice, or gluten-free pasta.

PER SERVING (4 to 5 scallops) Calories: 251;
Carbohydrates: 4g; Fat: 8g; Protein: 38g; Fiber: 0g;
Sodium: 445mg

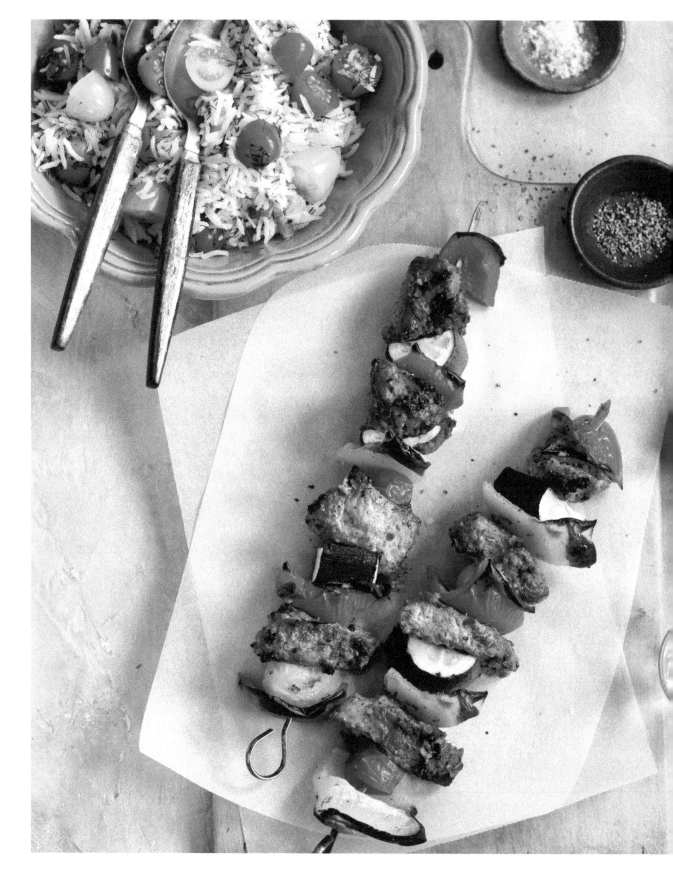

Chapter 9

Poultry

Left: Greek Chicken Kebabs

WHOLE ROASTED CHICKEN

Serves 5

PREP TIME: 45 MINUTES, PLUS 6 HOURS TO TENDERIZE / COOK TIME: 55 MINUTES

Whole roasted chicken always reminds me of Julia Child and her way of creating beautiful and sophisticated dishes for the everyday American meal. I would have loved to sit in her audience to see the magic with my own eyes. Roasted chicken doesn't have to be complicated to be sophisticated, nor does it have to be reserved only for special occasions. It can be made as a casual meal to brighten up a weeknight.

1 (3- to 3½-pound) whole chicken

Sea salt

Freshly ground black pepper

2 lemons, divided

3 tablespoons unsalted butter, at room temperature

2 tablespoons fresh oregano

2 tablespoons fresh rosemary

1. Line a baking sheet with parchment paper.

2. Pat the chicken dry with paper towels. Salt the entire chicken on the outside as well as inside the cavity. (This helps to tenderize the meat.)

3. Place the chicken on the baking sheet and refrigerate for at least 6 hours or overnight.

4. Pepper the entire chicken on the outside as well as inside the cavity.

5. Using a fork, pierce holes through the rind of 1 lemon. Place the pierced lemon inside the chicken cavity.

6. Rub the butter evenly over the skin of the chicken, then season it with more pepper.

7. Tightly tie the chicken legs together with kitchen twine. (This helps to ensure even cooking.)

8. Line a new rimmed baking sheet with parchment paper.

9. Slice the second lemon into ¼-inch rounds and place these in a single layer on the new rimmed baking sheet. Sprinkle with the oregano and rosemary.

10. Place the chicken on top of the lemon slices and herbs and let it sit for 30 minutes to come to room temperature.

11. While the chicken is sitting, preheat the oven to 450°F.

12. Roast the chicken for 20 minutes, then reduce the temperature to 350°F and continue roasting for 25 to 35 minutes, or until a food thermometer inserted into a breast and thigh reads 165°F.

13. Let the chicken rest for 10 minutes before carving.

MAKE-AHEAD TIP: A roasted chicken is great to make in the beginning of the week to have for salads, sandwiches, and entrées throughout the week. Store-bought rotisserie chickens usually have hidden FODMAP triggers like garlic and onion in their seasoning.

PER SERVING Calories: 271; Carbohydrates: 2g; Fat: 19g; Protein: 23g; Fiber: 1g; Sodium: 311mg

GREEK CHICKEN KEBABS

Serves 2

PREP TIME: 15 MINUTES, PLUS 30 MINUTES TO SOAK AND MARINATE / COOK TIME: 25 MINUTES

I grew up always wanting to help my parents in the kitchen. As a kid, being more involved with making dinner made it more satisfying to sit down and eat. Chicken kebabs are a great way to involve everyone. Young children especially love to skewer the chicken and vegetables and create their own custom kebabs. This recipe also works great with shrimp or beef instead of chicken. To fill out the meal, serve the kebabs alongside the Herbed Rice with Cherry Tomatoes (page 139).

1 tablespoon extra-virgin olive oil

1 tablespoon white wine vinegar

Juice of ½ lemon

1 tablespoon dried oregano

Zest of ½ lemon, plus additional for garnish (optional)

2 (4-ounce) boneless, skinless chicken breasts, cut into ½-inch cubes

Nonstick cooking spray

½ cup mixed yellow and red bell-pepper chunks

½ cup zucchini chunks

Sea salt

Freshly ground black pepper

1. Soak 2 wooden skewers in water for at least 30 minutes.

2. In a medium bowl, whisk together the olive oil, vinegar, lemon juice, oregano, and lemon zest (if using). Add the chicken, and stir to coat the cubes in the marinade. Cover the bowl and refrigerate for at least 30 minutes.

3. Preheat the oven to 400°F. Line a rimmed baking sheet with aluminum foil and spray it with the cooking spray.

4. Skewer the marinated chicken, bell pepper chunks, and zucchini chunks, and place the skewers on the baking sheet. Season them generously on both sides with salt and pepper.

5. Bake for 20 minutes, then turn the oven to broil and broil the kebabs for 2 minutes on each side, watching them carefully so they don't burn.

6. Garnish the kebabs with the lemon zest (if using).

PREP-AHEAD TIP: The chicken can be marinated overnight and skewered right before going into the oven.

PER SERVING (1 skewer) Calories: 218: Carbohydrates: 8g: Fat: 9g: Protein: 28g: Fiber: 3g: Sodium: 227mg

CHICKEN PICCATA

Serves 2

PREP TIME: 5 MINUTES / COOK TIME: 25 MINUTES

This is an impressive dish that anyone can make. I know this because my husband, who barely knows where the kitchen is in the house, has made this dish with no problems. In fact, it turned out perfectly! The key is to start with a pounded piece of chicken; this will help it cook through quickly and evenly.

2 (4-ounce) boneless, skinless chicken breasts, pounded to ¼-inch thickness

Sea salt

Freshly ground black pepper

¼ cup cornstarch

3 tablespoons unsalted butter

2 tablespoons brined capers

¼ cup white wine

Freshly squeezed lemon juice (optional)

1. Season the chicken on both sides with salt and pepper.

2. Put the cornstarch in a shallow bowl and lightly dredge both sides of the chicken breasts.

3. Melt the butter in a large skillet over medium-high heat. Add the chicken and cook for about 10 minutes on each side, until golden brown and cooked through. Transfer the chicken to a plate.

4. Reduce the heat to medium. Add the capers and wine to the pan and cook for about 3 minutes, stirring occasionally to scrape up any browned bits left from the chicken.

5. Remove the pan from the heat and pour the sauce over the chicken. Drizzle a squeeze of lemon juice (if using) over the chicken.

SERVING TIP: Serve over a bowl of gluten-free pasta or fresh sautéed spinach.

PER SERVING (1 breast) Calories: 358; Carbohydrates: 15g; Fat: 19g; Protein: 26g; Fiber: 0g; Sodium: 318mg

BAKED CHICKEN FAJITAS

Serves 2

PREP TIME: 10 MINUTES / COOK TIME: 20 MINUTES

I love ordering fajitas when we go out for Mexican food, but it can be nerve-racking trusting that there's no garlic or onion in the marinade. Most of the time, I choose not to order them. It's just not worth the risk of feeling sick and ruining the rest of the night. This recipe is delicious and FODMAP safe, using cumin, chili powder, and salt, with nary an onion or garlic clove in sight. Serve in corn tortillas or over rice, with a salad on the side.

Nonstick cooking spray

1 green bell pepper, sliced into ½-inch strips

1 red, yellow, or orange bell pepper, sliced into ½-inch strips

2 teaspoons ground chili powder

1 teaspoon sea salt

1 teaspoon ground cumin

4 (3-ounce) boneless, skinless chicken thighs

2 teaspoons extra-virgin olive oil

Juice of ½ lime

1. Preheat the oven to 400°F. Spray a 9-by-13-inch baking dish with the cooking spray.

2. To the baking dish, add the bell peppers, chili powder, salt, and cumin. Add the chicken, and use your hands to mix and coat the chicken with the spices. Drizzle the olive oil over the chicken.

3. Bake for 18 to 20 minutes, flipping the chicken over once, halfway through.

4. Drizzle the lime juice over the chicken and peppers.

INGREDIENT TIP: Top with fresh cilantro for an extra boost of flavor.

PER SERVING (2 chicken thighs) Calories: 261; Carbohydrates: 5g; Fat: 13g; Protein: 34g; Fiber: 2g; Sodium: 546mg

GROUND-CHICKEN MEATBALLS

Serves 4

PREP TIME: 10 MINUTES / COOK TIME: 20 MINUTES

Mamma meatballs! These meatballs are packed with flavor—and vegetables that even the most carnivorous eaters won't notice. If you're really daring, you can add shredded carrots for double the vegetables. I love eating these over Zoodles with Tomato Sauce (page 76), Summer Spaghetti Squash (page 81), gluten-free pasta, or rice.

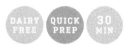

Nonstick cooking spray

½ cup shredded zucchini

1 pound ground chicken

1 egg

½ cup gluten-free bread crumbs

1 teaspoon dried oregano

Pinch sea salt

Freshly ground black pepper

SUBSTITUTION TIP: You can make these meatballs using ground turkey or beef instead of chicken.

MAKE-AHEAD TIP: Prepare the meatballs through step 4, then freeze them for 3 to 4 hours. Once frozen, store in a zip-top plastic bag and freeze for up to 3 to 4 months. Thaw completely before baking.

1. Preheat the oven to 400°F. Line a rimmed baking sheet with aluminum foil and spray it with the cooking spray.

2. Spread the shredded zucchini across a paper towel and cover it with a second paper towel. Press down to squeeze out the extra liquid.

3. Place the zucchini in a large bowl, and add the ground chicken, egg, bread crumbs, oregano, salt, and pepper. Use your hands to mix everything together until well combined.

4. Using your hands, roll the meat mixture into 2-inch-wide balls. Place the meatballs on the baking sheet, 2 inches apart.

5. Bake for 20 minutes, or until cooked through.

PER SERVING (3 to 5 meatballs) Calories: 198; Carbohydrates: 4g; Fat: 11g; Protein: 22g; Fiber: 1g; Sodium: 182mg

DAD'S EASY GRILLED CHICKEN

Serves 2

PREP TIME: 5 MINUTES / COOK TIME: 15 MINUTES

I grew up in a household of chicken dinners. We ate chicken at least five out of seven nights a week. To this day, I think my dad makes the best grilled chicken. There's no secret trick that I know of, except that he grills it with TLC (tender loving care). I always request this when we go to my parents' house for dinner because—as great as mine is—Dad's always tastes so much better.

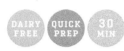

2 (4-ounce) boneless, skinless chicken breasts, pounded to ½-inch thickness

1 teaspoon salt

1 teaspoon freshly ground black pepper

1 teaspoon dried oregano

Extra-virgin olive oil

Nonstick cooking spray

1. Heat an outdoor grill or grill pan on medium-high heat for 10 to 15 minutes.

2. Season both sides of the chicken with the salt, pepper, and oregano. Drizzle it with olive oil.

3. Spray the cooking spray on the grill. Grill the chicken until cooked through, 6 to 7 minutes on each side.

MAKE-AHEAD TIP: Grilling chicken during your food prep can give you something to use in lunches and dinners for the upcoming week. Refrigerate in an airtight container for up to 1 week.

PER SERVING (1 chicken breast) Calories: 143; Carbohydrates: 1g; Fat: 4g; Protein: 26g; Fiber: 1g; Sodium: 1,238mg

PESTO-BAKED CHICKEN

Serves 2

PREP TIME: 5 MINUTES / COOK TIME: 25 MINUTES

Baked chicken recipes can be plain and boring. Using a flavorful marinade like pesto really amps up the flavors of the dish—plus the leftover pesto can be used for other meals later in the week. I like to make this meal when I'm in the mood for something quick but flavorful for dinner. There's definitely nothing boring about this chicken.

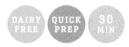

Nonstick cooking spray

Homemade Pesto (page 135)

2 (4-ounce) boneless, skinless
   chicken breasts

1. Preheat the oven to 400°F. Spray an 8-by-8-inch baking dish with the cooking spray.

2. Place the chicken breasts in the baking dish. Pour the pesto over the chicken and turn the breasts over so both sides are coated by the pesto.

3. Bake for 20 to 25 minutes, or until cooked through.

PREP-AHEAD TIP: The chicken can be marinated in the pesto overnight, too.

INGREDIENT TIP: Top the chicken with mozzarella cheese during the last 5 minutes of cooking.

PER SERVING (1 chicken breast [2 tablespoons pesto])
Calories: 182; Carbohydrates: 12g; Fat: 2g; Protein: 26g;
Fiber: 6g; Sodium: 1,004mg

LEMON AND HERB TURKEY CUTLETS

Serves 2

PREP TIME: 5 MINUTES / COOK TIME: 15 MINUTES

Turkey cutlets are a great alternative to chicken and cook in about the same amount of time. I've never been a fan of the traditional roasted turkey, as I find it to be dry and flavorless, but using turkey cutlets instead is a great way to maintain the flavor and juiciness of the meat. Just make sure to check the label on the chicken broth before you buy it—many store-bought broths contain FODMAP triggers like wheat, onion, and garlic.

2 (4-ounce) thinly sliced turkey cutlets

Pinch sea salt

Freshly ground black pepper

1 tablespoon extra-virgin olive oil

2 tablespoons unsalted butter

2 tablespoons chopped fresh herbs (such as rosemary, oregano, or sage)

½ cup low-sodium chicken broth (without garlic, onions, or celery)

Freshly squeezed lemon juice

1. Season the cutlets on both sides with salt and pepper.

2. Heat the olive oil in a large skillet over medium-high heat. Add the cutlets to the pan and cook until lightly browned and cooked through, about 5 minutes on each side. Transfer the turkey to a plate and set aside.

3. Lower the heat to medium-low and add the butter, herbs, and broth to the pan. Cook, stirring frequently, until the butter is fully melted, 1 to 2 minutes.

4. Return the cutlets to the pan and drizzle a squeeze of lemon juice over the turkey. Let it simmer for about 3 minutes before serving.

SUBSTITUTION TIP: Chicken or veal cutlets work great in this recipe as well.

PER SERVING (1 cutlet) Calories: 272; Carbohydrates: 5g; Fat: 19g; Protein: 21g; Fiber: 2g; Sodium: 525mg

TURKEY TACOS

Serves 4

PREP TIME: 5 MINUTES / COOK TIME: 25 MINUTES

Taco Tuesday has practically become a national pastime, and I fully support having tacos any day of the week. There are also many uses for this seasoned ground turkey beyond tacos, like salads, rice bowls, and quesadillas.

Nonstick cooking spray

1 tablespoon chopped scallions

1 pound ground turkey

½ teaspoon ground cumin

1½ teaspoons chili powder

Pinch sea salt

Freshly ground black pepper

1. Spray a large skillet with the cooking spray and place it over medium heat. Add the scallions and sauté until softened, 1 to 2 minutes.

2. Add the ground turkey and begin to brown it, using a wooden spoon to break it apart into crumbles. Brown and break apart the meat for about 3 minutes.

3. Stir in the cumin and chili powder, and season with salt and pepper. Continue to cook the meat until it's browned and cooked through, 15 to 20 minutes.

SERVING TIP: Serve with corn tortillas and FODMAP-safe taco fixin's like shredded lettuce and diced tomatoes.

PER SERVING (½ cup) Calories: 131; Carbohydrates: 1g; Fat: 3g; Protein: 27g; Fiber: 0g; Sodium: 106mg

CLASSIC TURKEY BURGERS

Serves 4

PREP TIME: 10 MINUTES, PLUS 30 TO 60 MINUTES TO FIRM / COOK TIME: 12 MINUTES

Sometimes I crave a hearty turkey burger, but it can be hard to order one when eating out due to the premixed bread crumbs, garlic, and onions that are usually included. After my last burger craving, I created this classic recipe, rich in flavor but without the hidden FODMAP triggers. I know these will be a hit at your next barbecue or family gathering.

1 pound ground turkey

¼ cup gluten-free bread crumbs

1 egg white

2 tablespoons soy sauce

2 tablespoons chopped scallions

1 tablespoon dried oregano

Pinch sea salt

Freshly ground black pepper

Nonstick cooking spray

PREP-AHEAD TIP: The patties can be made the night before and kept in an airtight container in the refrigerator until ready to cook.

1. In a large bowl, add the ground turkey, bread crumbs, egg white, soy sauce, scallions, and oregano, and season with salt and pepper. Using your hands, mix everything together until well combined.

2. Divide the mixture into 4 equal portions and form each into a ball about 3 inches wide. Gently flatten the ball to create a patty about ½ inch thick. For the best results, refrigerate the patties for 30 minutes to 1 hour, to let them firm up.

3. Spray a large skillet with the cooking spray and place it over medium-high heat. Once hot, add each patty to the pan and cook until browned and cooked through, about 6 minutes on each side.

PER SERVING (1 burger) Calories: 143; Carbohydrates: 3g; Fat: 3g; Protein: 28g; Fiber: 1g; Sodium: 574mg

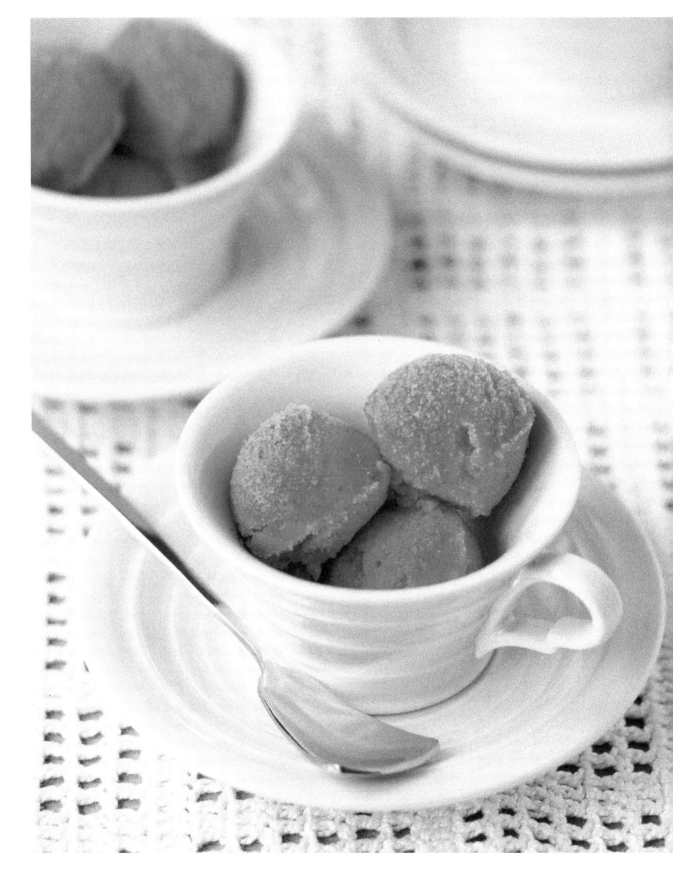

Chapter 10

Snacks and Desserts

Left: Berry Berry Sorbet

PEANUT-BUTTER ENERGY BALLS

Makes 24 balls

PREP TIME: 10 MINUTES, PLUS 1 HOUR TO CHILL

It can be hard to find FODMAP-safe snacks to grab and go, which is why I'm obsessed with these energy balls. These have all the workings of a perfect protein snack, including oats and peanut butter, and the chocolate chips add a touch of sweetness. What else could you want? The best part is that they can be made in advance and refrigerated for when you need a boost of extra energy.

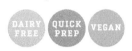

1½ cups steel-cut oats

½ cup peanut butter or other nut butter

¼ cup maple syrup

1 teaspoon ground cinnamon

¼ teaspoon sea salt

2 tablespoons dark-chocolate chips

1. Line a baking sheet with waxed paper.

2. To the bowl of a food processor, add the oats, peanut butter, maple syrup, cinnamon, and salt. Pulse just until the ingredients are mixed together. Add the chocolate chips and pulse until the chips are pulverized and the mixture has achieved a sticky texture.

3. Using wet hands, form the mixture into 1-inch-wide balls. Place them on the baking sheet.

4. Refrigerate the energy balls for at least 1 hour so they firm up. Then store in an airtight container in the refrigerator for up to 1 week.

SUBSTITUTION TIP: You can use almond butter, ¼ cup of shredded coconut, chia seeds, and/or hemp seeds to create different varieties.

PER SERVING (1 ball) Calories: 53; Carbohydrates: 5g; Fat: 3g; Protein: 2g; Fiber: 1g; Sodium: 45mg

BANANA-BREAD MUFFINS

Makes 12 muffins

PREP TIME: 15 MINUTES / COOK TIME: 30 MINUTES

I love all things banana bread, and this recipe is no exception. It makes for a perfect breakfast, snack, or dessert. I love using muffin tins instead of a bread pan—that way, the muffins are already portioned out and no slicing is needed. Sometimes I also double the recipe and freeze some of the muffins for when guests come over or when I need a last-minute homemade gift.

2 cups oat flour

1 teaspoon baking soda

Pinch sea salt

1 tablespoon ground cinnamon

½ cup coconut oil

3 unripe bananas, mashed

2 eggs

¾ cup raw sugar

¼ cup maple syrup

½ teaspoon pure vanilla extract

½ cup chopped walnuts or pecans

½ cup blueberries

1. Preheat the oven to 325°F. Line a muffin tin with paper liners.

2. Combine the oat flour, baking soda, salt, and cinnamon in a medium bowl. Set aside.

3. In a small microwave-safe bowl, melt the coconut oil in the microwave. Pour it into a large mixing bowl and add the mashed bananas, eggs, sugar, maple syrup, and vanilla. Mix well.

4. Add the dry ingredients to the wet ingredients, and stir until well combined. Gently fold in the walnuts and blueberries.

5. Fill each muffin cup three-quarters full. Bake for 25 to 30 minutes, or until a toothpick inserted into the center of a muffin comes out clean.

ALLERGEN TIP: The nuts can be omitted completely or substituted with pumpkin seeds or sunflower seeds.

PER SERVING (1 muffin) Calories: 213; Carbohydrates: 29g; Fat: 11g; Protein: 2g; Fiber: 2g; Sodium: 135mg

BERRY FRUIT LEATHERS

Makes 16 leathers

PREP TIME: 5 MINUTES / COOK TIME: 3 TO 3½ HOURS

When I was growing up, my house was the place to go for junk food. Everyone's favorite was the fruity snacks that were high in sugar and low in fruit. This fruit leather recipe is in honor of my beloved childhood snack—but this version is made from actual fruit and natural sugars. The hardest part of the whole recipe is being patient enough to wait for the leathers to bake in the oven.

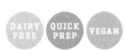

2 cups strawberries

2 cups blueberries

½ cup maple syrup

Juice of 1 lemon

1. Preheat the oven to 200°F. Line two baking sheets with parchment paper.

2. Add the strawberries, blueberries, maple syrup, and lemon juice to a blender, and blend until smooth.

3. Divide the mixture between the two small baking sheets and use a rubber spatula to spread it across the sheets in an even layer.

4. Bake for 3 to 3½ hours, or until no longer sticky when you tap it with your finger.

5. Let the berry leather cool for about 30 minutes, then use a pizza cutter or scissors to cut it into 8 strips, each about 1 inch wide and 5 inches long.

MAKE-AHEAD TIP: These can be stored in an airtight container in your pantry for up to 3 weeks.

PER SERVING (1 leather) Calories: 38; Carbohydrates: 11g; Fat: 0g; Protein: 0.5g; Fiber: 1g; Sodium: 2mg

CHOCOLATE-COVERED BANANA SLICES

Serves 1 to 2

PREP TIME: 10 MINUTES, PLUS 1 HOUR TO CHILL / COOK TIME: 5 MINUTES

This is a great quick dessert to whip up when you want a sweet treat but don't want to majorly splurge or spend a lot of time putting something together. Plus, you can never go wrong with chocolate-dipped anything. Feel free to use any low-FODMAP fruit you have available. I like orange slices and strawberries dipped in chocolate, too.

1 unripe banana, frozen and sliced

½ cup high-quality milk- or dark-chocolate chips

1. Line a baking sheet with parchment paper and place the banana slices on the sheet in a single layer so that they're not touching each other.

2. In a microwave-safe bowl, melt the chocolate in the microwave at 30-second intervals, making sure to stir it between intervals.

3. Pour the chocolate over the banana slices so they're completely covered.

4. Refrigerate for at least 1 hour so the chocolate hardens completely. Transfer to an airtight container and refrigerate for up to 1 week.

MAKE-AHEAD TIP: I always have these handy in the freezer for when I need a "bite" of chocolate to satisfy my craving. Store in a zip-top plastic bag or freezer-safe container for up to 3 months.

PER SERVING (½ banana) Calories: 333; Carbohydrates: 46g; Fat: 20g; Protein: 5g; Fiber: 6g; Sodium: 1mg

COCONUT MACAROONS

Makes 24 macaroons

PREP TIME: 10 MINUTES / COOK TIME: 15 MINUTES

Macaroons are the perfect low-FODMAP, gluten-free (and Passover-friendly!) dessert that can be made any time of the year. This recipe is so much better than any packaged version you can find in the stores. These make for an excellent grab-and-go snack as well.

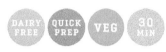

6 egg whites

Pinch sea salt

½ cup maple syrup

1 tablespoon vanilla extract

3 cups unsweetened shredded coconut

1. Preheat the oven to 350°F. Line two baking sheets with parchment paper.

2. In a small bowl, add the egg whites and salt. Using an electric mixer on high speed, whisk the eggs until firm peaks form, 5 to 6 minutes.

3. Using a rubber spatula, gently fold in the maple syrup, vanilla, and coconut until well combined.

4. Drop 1 rounded tablespoon of batter at a time on the baking sheet, leaving about 2 inches between each macaroon.

5. Bake for 12 to 15 minutes, or until lightly browned.

BAKING TIP: These can be sticky when they first come out of the oven. Make sure to let them sit for 10 to 15 minutes before transferring to a cooling rack.

PER SERVING (2 macaroons) Calories: 156; Carbohydrates: 13g; Fat: 10g; Protein: 3g; Fiber: 2g; Sodium: 42mg

ROASTED EGGPLANT DIP

Makes 2 cups

PREP TIME: 20 MINUTES / COOK TIME: 25 MINUTES

Eggplant is low–FODMAP, low in calories, and high in antioxidants, which makes it a great choice to cook with. I love all things ending in "dip," and this recipe is no exception. Mediterranean dips like Hummus (page 136) and eggplant dip are delicious and satisfying snacks, but store–bought varieties are usually heavy in garlic, or contain larger quantities of tahini sauce and chickpeas. So I created my own!

1 large eggplant

2 tablespoons peanut butter or nut butter

Juice of 1 lemon, plus additional if needed

¼ cup extra-virgin olive oil

Kosher salt

1. Preheat the oven to 400°F. Line a baking sheet with parchment paper.

2. Prick the eggplant all over with a fork and place it on the baking sheet. Bake for about 25 minutes, until the skin begins to brown and blister. Set aside until cool enough to touch (about 15 minutes).

3. Halve the eggplant. Using a spoon, scoop the soft flesh out of the eggplant and into the bowl of a food processor.

4. Add the peanut butter, lemon juice, olive oil, and salt to the food processor, and process until smooth, 1 to 2 minutes. Taste, and season with additional salt or lemon, if needed.

SERVING TIP: Serve this dip with carrots, endive, and/or gluten-free crackers.

PER SERVING (2 tablespoons) Calories: 60; Carbohydrates: 3g; Fat: 5g; Protein: 1g; Fiber: 2g; Sodium: 31mg

BANANA ICE CREAM

Makes 2 cups

PREP TIME: 5 MINUTES

Banana ice cream is one of my all-time favorite desserts to make, and it takes less than 5 minutes to whip up. I like to have a batch in the freezer at all times for when a craving hits. The consistency and taste is just like ice cream made with dairy, but without the lactose.

2 frozen bananas

2 tablespoons cocoa powder

2 tablespoons peanut butter

1 teaspoon maple syrup

½ teaspoon vanilla extract

Put the frozen bananas, cocoa powder, peanut butter, maple syrup, and vanilla in a blender, and blend until smooth. Serve immediately or freeze in an airtight, freezer-safe container.

INGREDIENT TIP: You can include any number of low-FODMAP add-ins, such as cinnamon, cacao nibs, or fresh mint, for fun variations.

PER SERVING (½ cup) Calories: 111; Carbohydrates: 18g; Fat: 5g; Protein: 3g; Fiber: 3g; Sodium: 38mg

BERRY BERRY SORBET

Makes 2 cups

PREP TIME: 30 MINUTES, PLUS 2 HOURS TO FREEZE

Sorbet is one of my favorite desserts. It's the perfect way to combat the summer heat, and with this recipe, you can feel good knowing you're eating a healthy dessert made from pure fruit. You won't believe how satisfying this homemade treat is—and you definitely won't feel any guilt going for a second scoop of it.

1 cup halved strawberries

1 cup blueberries

Juice of 1 lemon

⅓ cup maple syrup

1. In a blender, add the strawberries, blueberries, lemon juice, and maple syrup. Blend until the mixture has a smooth and even texture.

2. Pour the mixture into an ice cream maker and freeze the sorbet according to the manufacturer's instructions. It takes about 25 minutes.

3. Transfer the sorbet into an airtight, freezer-safe container and let freeze for at least 2 hours before serving.

SUBSTITUTION TIP: This is a basic sorbet recipe that can be substituted with any other low-FODMAP fruit like honeydew or pineapple.

PER SERVING (½ cup) Calories: 104; Carbohydrates: 26g; Fat: 0g; Protein: 1g; Fiber: 2g; Sodium: 5mg

OATMEAL SEMISWEET CHOCOLATE-CHIP COOKIES

Makes 24 cookies

PREP TIME: 15 MINUTES / COOK TIME: 11 MINUTES

Call me plain Jane, but my all-time favorite dessert is a simple chocolate-chip cookie. This was my number-one concern when I eliminated gluten from my diet: Would I still be able to make a winning chocolate-chip cookie? With this recipe, the answer is yes! And if you have one for breakfast, who am I to judge? They do have oats in them, after all.

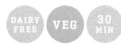

2½ cups oat flour

1 teaspoon baking soda

Pinch sea salt, plus extra for garnish

½ cup coconut oil

⅔ cup dark brown sugar

1 egg

1 teaspoon vanilla extract

½ cup semisweet chocolate chips

1. Preheat the oven to 350°F. Line two baking sheets with parchment paper.

2. In a medium bowl, combine the oat flour, baking soda, and salt. Set aside.

3. In a microwave-safe bowl, melt the coconut oil in a microwave, then pour it into a large mixing bowl.

4. To this large bowl, add the sugar, egg, and vanilla. Mix until well combined.

5. Add the dry ingredients to the wet ingredients and mix well.

6. Fold in the chocolate chips until just combined.

7. Put tablespoon-size scoops of batter on the baking sheets, leaving about 2 inches between each cookie. Bake for about 11 minutes, or until golden brown.

8. As soon as the cookies come out of the oven, sprinkle them with a little salt. Let the cookies cool on the pan for about 2 minutes, then transfer them to a wire rack to cool completely.

SUBSTITUTION TIP: Feel free to use a different oil if you don't have any coconut oil available.

PER SERVING (1 cookie) Calories: 93; Carbohydrates: 9g; Fat: 6g; Protein: 1g; Fiber: 1g; Sodium: 67mg

COCONUT-LEMON BARS

Makes 12 bars

PREP TIME: 40 MINUTES / COOK TIME: 32 MINUTES, PLUS 1 HOUR TO CHILL

These lemon bars are a labor of love with three separate parts to make: the crust, the filling, and the topping. But the extra time is more than worth it when you take that first bite of the bar. It's important to use fresh lemons rather than lemon concentrate in order to get the freshest flavor in each sweet, tart bite.

FOR THE CRUST

Nonstick cooking spray

1½ cups old-fashioned oats

½ cup unsweetened shredded coconut

¼ cup raw sugar

Pinch sea salt

¼ cup coconut oil

FOR THE FILLING

2 eggs

½ cup raw sugar

5 tablespoons freshly squeezed lemon juice

1 tablespoon freshly grated lemon zest

1 teaspoon vanilla extract

2 tablespoons cornstarch

FOR THE TOPPING

⅓ cup raw sugar

¼ cup freshly squeezed lemon juice

¼ cup water

2 tablespoons cornstarch

¼ cup unsweetened shredded coconut

TO MAKE THE CRUST

1. Preheat the oven to 350°F. Spray an 8-by-8-inch baking pan with the cooking spray.

2. In a food processor, add the oats, coconut, and sugar. Process until they're combined and ground to a fine texture.

3. In a microwafe-safe bowl, melt the coconut oil in a microwave. Add the melted coconut oil to the food processor, and pulse until it's combined with the oat mixture.

4. Transfer the mixture to the baking pan and press it down with the back of a spoon until it covers the bottom of the pan in an even layer.

5. Bake for about 14 minutes, or until golden brown. Set aside to cool for at least 20 minutes.

TO MAKE THE FILLING

1. While the crust is cooling, add the eggs to the bowl of a stand mixer. Beat on medium-high speed for 2 to 3 minutes, until the eggs are light and foamy.

2. Add the sugar, lemon juice, lemon zest, and vanilla, and continue mixing until completely combined, about 1 minute.

3. Put ¼ cup of the egg mixture in a small bowl and whisk in the cornstarch. Add that back into the bowl of the stand mixer, and whisk well until fully incorporated.

4. Pour the filling into the cooled crust. Bake for 18 minutes, or until the top is no longer wet.

TO MAKE THE TOPPING

1. While the filling and crust are baking, in a small saucepan over medium heat, add the sugar, lemon juice, water, and cornstarch. Heat, stirring frequently, until the mixture thickens, 2 to 3 minutes. Stir in the coconut and remove the pan from the heat.

2. Pour the topping over the baked lemon bars and gently spread it across into an even layer.

3. Chill the pan in the refrigerator for at least 1 hour before slicing.

INGREDIENT TIP: These are especially delicious with Coconut Whipped Cream (page 132) served on top.

PER SERVING (1 bar) Calories: 251; Carbohydrates: 30g; Fat: 14g; Protein: 3g; Fiber: 3g; Sodium: 37mg

FLOURLESS CHOCOLATE CAKE WITH BERRY SAUCE

Serves 10

PREP TIME: 20 MINUTES / COOK TIME: 30 MINUTES

My family is chocolate obsessed, and I knew this recipe would be a huge hit the first time I made it. The berry sauce adds a touch of light, tart sweetness, which perfectly complements the velvety richness of the cake. This cake is naturally gluten-free, and no one will miss the wheat for a second.

FOR THE CAKE

½ cup (or 1 stick) unsalted butter, chopped, plus additional for greasing the pan

6 ounces dark chocolate, chopped

2 egg whites

¾ cup white sugar

3 eggs

½ cup high-quality unsweetened cocoa powder, sifted

FOR THE BERRY SAUCE

2 cups frozen strawberries

2 cups blueberries

⅓ cup maple syrup

2 tablespoons freshly squeezed lemon juice

TO MAKE THE CAKE

1. Preheat the oven to 350°F.

2. Grease the bottom and sides of a 9-inch round cake pan with butter, line the bottom of the pan with parchment paper, and grease the top of the paper with more butter.

3. Using a double boiler or a heatproof bowl nestled over a pot of boiling water, melt the chocolate and ½ cup of butter until smooth, stirring frequently. Remove from the heat and set aside.

4. Using an electric mixer, beat the egg whites on medium-high speed until soft peaks form, about 3 minutes. With the mixer running, slowly add the sugar, and mix until just combined.

5. In a large bowl, whisk together the eggs and cocoa powder until just combined.

6. Pour the melted-chocolate mixture into the egg mixture and stir to combine. Then gently fold the egg whites into the batter until just combined, making sure not to overmix. Pour the batter into the cake pan.

7. Bake for about 30 minutes, rotating the pan once after 15 minutes. The cake is ready once it's set in the center and begins to pull away from the sides of the pan. Let the cake cool completely before removing it from the pan.

TO MAKE THE BERRY SAUCE

1. Put the strawberries, blueberries, maple syrup, and lemon juice in a medium saucepan over medium-high heat. Use the back of a spoon to break down the berries into smaller pieces as they heat. Constantly stir the sauce until it begins to bubble and thicken, 2 to 3 minutes.

2. Remove the saucepan from the heat and let the sauce cool before serving.

INGREDIENT TIP: Splurge on buying high-quality dark chocolate. You'll notice a difference in the taste and quality of the cake. Also, you can use fresh strawberries instead of frozen when making the sauce. Just add ¼ cup of water to the saucepan with the other ingredients.

PER SERVING (1 slice) Calories: 296; Carbohydrates: 42g; Fat: 16g; Protein: 5g; Fiber: 4g; Sodium: 37mg

BAKED PARSNIP CHIPS

Serves 4

PREP TIME: 5 MINUTES / COOK TIME: 30 MINUTES

Root-vegetable chips are a great alternative to potato chips and just as addictive. I dare you to eat just one. This recipe works with other low-FODMAP vegetables like potatoes (yes, you can make your own potato chips!), carrots, and zucchini. These chips are not fried, which makes them easier on sensitive stomachs.

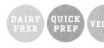

3 parsnips
½ teaspoon extra-virgin olive oil
Pinch sea salt
Freshly ground black pepper

1. Preheat the oven to 375°F. Line a baking sheet with parchment paper.

2. Using the slicing blade of a food processor (or a mandoline slicer), thinly slice the parsnips, leaving the skin on.

3. In a large bowl, gently mix the sliced parsnips, olive oil, salt, and pepper, until the slices are coated on both sides.

4. Place the parsnip slices in an even layer on the baking sheet, making sure they don't overlap. Bake for 15 minutes, flip over the chips, and bake for 15 minutes more, or until golden brown and crispy.

INGREDIENT TIP: These chips are perfect to dip in the Roasted Eggplant Dip (page 117) or Hummus (page 136).

PER SERVING (½ cup) Calories: 79; Carbohydrates: 18g; Fat: 1g; Protein: 1g; Fiber: 5g; Sodium: 49mg

GRANDMA'S FRUIT SALAD

Serves 8

PREP TIME: 10 MINUTES

I grew up visiting my grandparents in Memphis, Tennessee, every summer, and we ate my grandma's special fruit salad before every dinner. It always felt like such a treat being served fruit salad in a pretty bowl. I later learned that the secret ingredient that kept the fruit fresh and vibrant was a dash of orange juice.

2 unripe bananas, sliced

2 cups sliced strawberries

2 cups blueberries

2 teaspoons freshly squeezed orange juice

Fresh mint leaves (optional)

1. Combine the bananas, strawberries, blueberries, and orange juice in a large bowl.

2. Refrigerate until ready to serve. Garnish with the mint leaves (if using).

SUBSTITUTION TIP: Other low-FODMAP fruits, like orange slices, honeydew, or cantaloupe, can be used in place of the berries and bananas.

PAIRING TIP: Along with the fruit, enjoy protein-rich, low-FODMAP hard cheese or lactose-free yogurt to improve fructose absorption.

PER SERVING (½ cup) Calories: 61; Carbohydrates: 15g; Fat: 0g; Protein: 1g; Fiber: 3g; Sodium: 1mg

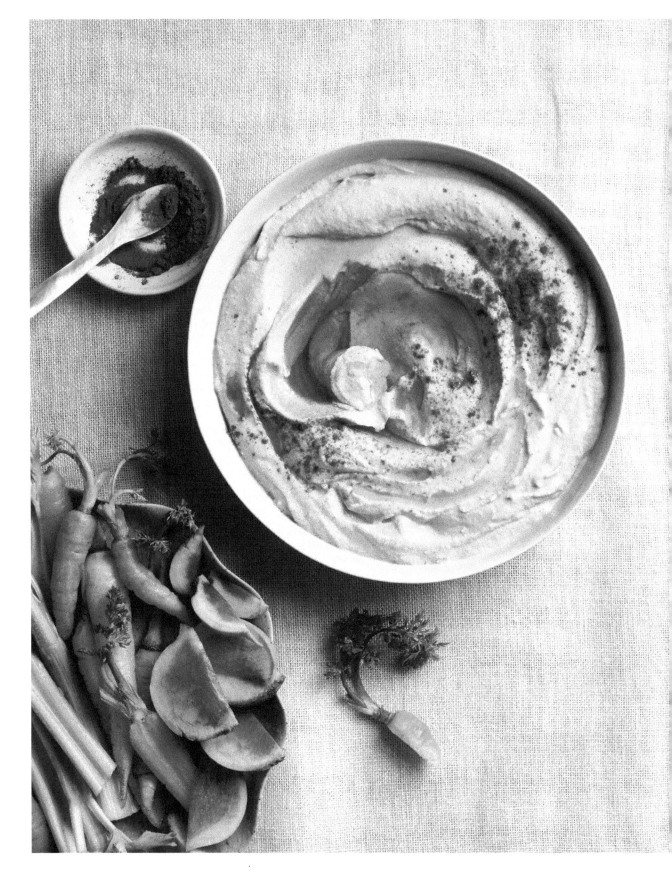

Kitchen Staples

Left: Hummus

BASIC VINAIGRETTE

Makes 1 cup

PREP TIME: 5 MINUTES

Salad dressing is unbelievably easy to make and tastes so much better than anything you buy at the store. Plus, I love impressing my guests by being able to say I made it myself. Just shake it before each use and take your salad to the next level.

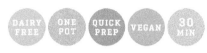

¾ cup extra virgin olive oil

¼ cup balsamic vinegar

1 teaspoon Dijon mustard

Pinch sea salt

Freshly ground black pepper

In a mason jar or other container with an airtight lid, add the olive oil, balsamic vinegar, mustard, salt, and pepper, and shake well.

MAKE-AHEAD TIP: This can be kept in the refrigerator for up to 2 weeks. Shake the dressing well before each use.

PER SERVING (2 tablespoons) Calories: 167;
Carbohydrates: 1g; Fat: 19g; Protein: 1g; Fiber: 0g;
Sodium: 27mg

ITALIAN SALAD DRESSING

Makes 1 cup

PREP TIME: 5 MINUTES

Italian salad dressing is another classic dressing that typically has garlic and onion in it, making it one to avoid both in the grocery store and when eating out. This low–FODMAP version is another crowd pleaser to have on hand.

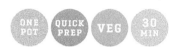

¾ cup extra-virgin olive oil

¼ cup red-wine vinegar

2 tablespoons Parmesan cheese

1 teaspoon dried oregano

Sea salt

Freshly ground black pepper

In a mason jar or other container with an airtight lid, add the olive oil, vinegar, cheese, oregano, salt, and pepper, and shake well.

MAKE-AHEAD TIP: This can be kept in the refrigerator for up to 2 weeks. Shake the dressing well before each use.

PER SERVING (2 tablespoons) Calories: 169; Carbohydrates: 0g; Fat: 19g; Protein: 1g; Fiber: 0g; Sodium: 53mg

COCONUT WHIPPED CREAM

Makes 2 cups

PREP TIME: 10 MINUTES

Once you make whipped cream at home, you'll never want store-bought again. Whipped cream is delicious over just about anything. I love to add a dollop to a bowl of fruit or on a slice of cake. Serve this with Coconut-Lemon Bars (page 122) for an out-of-this-world dessert.

1 (14-ounce) can coconut cream

¼ cup powdered sugar

1 teaspoon maple syrup

½ teaspoon vanilla extract

1. Use a spoon to remove only the top layer of white cream off the top of the coconut cream, making sure to avoid the coconut water. Place the cream in a large bowl.

2. Add the powdered sugar, maple syrup, and vanilla to the bowl. Using an electric mixer, whip the ingredients on high speed until soft peaks form, 2 to 3 minutes.

INGREDIENT TIP: Refrigerate the can of coconut cream overnight to help "set" or separate the cream from the water. Make sure not to shake the can before you open it.

PER SERVING (½ cup) Calories: 511; Carbohydrates: 80g; Fat: 22g; Protein: 2g; Fiber: 0g; Sodium: 48mg

SUN-DRIED TOMATOES

Makes 2 cups

PREP TIME: 5 MINUTES / COOK TIME: 5 HOURS

I can never eat cherry tomatoes fast enough before they go bad. To solve this problem, I started making my own sun-dried tomatoes. Not only are these substantially cheaper than anything you can find in the store, they're also dried without being soaked in oil. I love using them as a great flavor booster to add to pasta, chicken dishes, and salads.

2 cups cherry tomatoes, sliced lengthwise

Sea salt

1. Preheat the oven to 200°F. Line a baking sheet with parchment paper.

2. Place the sliced tomatoes cut-side up on the baking sheet. Lightly pat them dry with a paper towel. Sprinkle them with some salt.

3. Bake for 5 hours, or until dried and wrinkled.

MAKE-AHEAD TIP: Store in an airtight container in the refrigerator for up to 3 weeks.

PER SERVING (1 tablespoon) Calories: 2; Carbohydrates: 0g; Fat: 0g; Protein: 0g; Fiber: 0g; Sodium: 8g

HOMEMADE KETCHUP

Makes 2 cups

PREP TIME: 5 MINUTES / COOK TIME: 20 MINUTES

I was shocked to find out how many FODMAP triggers like high-fructose corn syrup and onion powder are hidden in most store-bought ketchups. This homemade version is 100 percent FODMAP safe and tastes absolutely delicious. Adding to its star power, it takes very little time to make.

2 (6-ounce) cans tomato paste

1 cup water

¼ cup apple cider vinegar

¼ cup maple syrup

1 tablespoon raw sugar

2 teaspoons sea salt

1. In a medium saucepan over medium heat, whisk together the tomato paste, water, vinegar, maple syrup, sugar, and salt until the sauce begins to boil.

2. Reduce the heat to a simmer and cook, stirring constantly, for 15 to 20 minutes.

MAKE-AHEAD TIP: This ketchup will last in an airtight container for up to 1 month. Ketch-up later!

PER SERVING (1 tablespoon) Calories: 17; Carbohydrates: 4g; Fat: 0g; Protein: 1g; Fiber: 0g; Sodium: 128mg

HOMEMADE PESTO

Makes ½ cup

PREP TIME: 5 MINUTES

Store-bought pesto is always so expensive and, of course, made with garlic. The first time I made this garlic-free version for myself, I knew I'd never buy it premade again. My version comes together in under 3 minutes and is packed with so much fresh basil flavor.

DAIRY FREE · ONE POT · QUICK PREP · VEGAN · 30 MIN

1 cup packed basil

5 tablespoons extra-virgin olive oil or garlic-infused olive oil

2 tablespoons walnuts or other low-FODMAP nut or seed of your choice

2 tablespoons nutritional yeast

Pinch sea salt

In a food processor, combine the basil, olive oil, walnuts, nutritional yeast, and salt, and process until it forms a paste-like consistency, about 3 minutes.

MAKE-AHEAD TIP: This can be made in advance and kept in the refrigerator for up to 1 week.

INGREDIENT TIP: Avoid swapping the walnuts for cashews or pistachios, since these are high-FODMAP.

PER SERVING (1 tablespoon) Calories: 100; Carbohydrates: 2g; Fat: 10g; Protein: 2g; Fiber: 1g; Sodium: 33mg

HUMMUS

Makes 1 cup

PREP TIME: 10 MINUTES

Hummus is a great source of protein and makes for a perfectly healthy snack to go along with vegetables and crackers. According to a Monash University study, chickpeas are considered low-FODMAP based on a ¼-cup serving size. Once the portion increases to ½ cup, you're in the moderate category for galactans.

1 (15-ounce) can chickpeas, drained and rinsed

2 tablespoons extra-virgin olive oil, plus additional if needed

1 teaspoon fine sea salt

Freshly ground black pepper

1 tablespoon tahini (no more)

Juice of ½ lemon

½ teaspoon maple syrup

2 tablespoons water, plus additional if needed

Paprika, for garnish (optional)

1. In a food processor, add the chickpeas, olive oil, salt, pepper, tahini, lemon juice, maple syrup, and water. Process until the hummus is smooth, about 3 minutes. If it's too thick, or you prefer a thinner hummus, add more water and olive oil as needed to reach your preferred consistency.

2. Transfer to a bowl and garnish with the paprika (if using).

INGREDIENT TIP: Experiment with adding fresh herbs like basil and cilantro to change up the flavor profile.

PER SERVING (2 tablespoons) Calories: 103; Carbohydrates: 14g; Fat: 4g; Protein: 3g; Fiber: 3g; Sodium: 414mg

EASY PASTA SAUCE

Serves 4

PREP TIME: 5 MINUTES

It is close to impossible to find a store-bought pasta sauce that is garlic- and onion-free. That's why I came up with this 5-minute pasta sauce that tastes like you slaved in the kitchen for hours to make it. It really only takes a few quality ingredients to make a gourmet sauce.

5 medium tomatoes, chopped

1 cup loosely packed basil

⅓ cup extra-virgin olive oil or garlic-infused olive oil

¼ cup Sun-Dried Tomatoes (page 133)

¼ cup tomato paste

Pinch sea salt, plus more for seasoning

Freshly ground black pepper

Add the tomatoes, basil, olive oil, sun-dried tomatoes, tomato paste, salt, and pepper to a food processor, and process to your desired consistency. If needed, add more salt.

MAKE-AHEAD TIP: This pasta sauce can be made in advance and stored in the freezer in an airtight container for up to 2 months.

INGREDIENT TIP: Stick closely to the recommended amount of sun-dried tomatoes. A higher portion will contain more fructans, which may be uncomfortable for your digestive system.

PER SERVING (½ cup) Calories: 194; Carbohydrates: 11g; Fat: 3g; Protein: 3g; Fiber: 3g; Sodium: 133mg

FOOLPROOF QUINOA

Serves 4

PREP TIME: 1 MINUTE / COOK TIME: 20 MINUTES

Some people are unfamiliar with this grain (technically, it's a seed), but it has actually been around for more than 3,000 years. Quinoa is one of my favorite naturally gluten-free, low-FODMAP grains to use for cooking. It has amazing versatility and health benefits, such as being high in protein and fiber. Use it just as you would rice or any other grain. Bonus points that quinoa cooks quicker than rice!

2 cups water

1 cup quinoa

Pinch sea salt

1. In a medium saucepan, bring the water, quinoa, and salt to a boil.

2. Cover the pan, reduce the heat to low, and cook for 15 minutes, or until the quinoa is tender and all the water is absorbed.

3. Remove the pan from the heat and fluff the quinoa with a fork. Cover the top of the quinoa with a paper towel and put the lid back on the pan. Let the quinoa sit for 5 minutes. This is my secret to getting the fluffiest quinoa.

MAKE-AHEAD TIP: A batch of quinoa can be made ahead of time and eaten all week. Just refrigerate in an airtight container.

PER SERVING (½ cup) Calories: 157; Carbohydrates: 27g; Fat: 3g; Protein: 6g; Fiber: 3g; Sodium: 41mg

HERBED RICE WITH CHERRY TOMATOES

Serves 4

PREP TIME: 5 MINUTES / COOK TIME: 20 MINUTES

Rice is definitely one of my comfort foods. For me, there's nothing more soothing than a bowl of rice. But sometimes I want to ramp up the flavor, and the easiest way to do that is by substituting broth for water and adding some bold herbs. This side dish is a perfect accompaniment for chicken and seafood recipes.

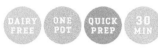

1 cup basmati rice

1 cup water

¾ cup chicken or vegetable broth

1 teaspoon salt

1 cup cherry tomatoes, halved

2 tablespoons fresh dill

2 tablespoons fresh parsley

1. In a medium saucepan, bring the rice, water, broth, and salt to boil.

2. Cover the pan and reduce the heat to low. Cook for 15 minutes, or until the rice is tender and the water is absorbed.

3. Remove the pan from the heat and fluff the rice with a fork. Stir in the cherry tomatoes, dill, and parsley. Cover the top of the rice with a paper towel and put the lid back on the pan. Let the rice sit for 5 minutes.

INGREDIENT TIP: If you don't have fresh herbs available, just use half the amount of dried herbs.

PER SERVING (½ cup) Calories: 189; Carbohydrates: 40g; Fat: 1g; Protein: 5g; Fiber: 1g; Sodium: 733mg

HOMEMADE ALMOND BUTTER

Makes 1 cup

PREP TIME: 7 MINUTES

I grew up eating peanut butter and jelly sandwiches every single day for my school lunch. I still think there's nothing more satisfying than a good PB&J, but these days mine are a little bit more gourmet. The taste of homemade nut butter has much more richness and flavor than any store-bought version, plus it's a great cost saver in the long run. With my Strawberry Jam (page 141), it's a slam dunk.

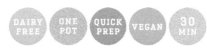

2 cups raw almonds

½ teaspoon sea salt

1 tablespoon ground cinnamon (optional)

In a food processor, combine the almonds, salt, and cinnamon (if using), and process for 5 to 7 minutes, scraping down the sides of the bowl about every 2 minutes, until a butter-like consistency forms.

ALLERGEN TIP: You can substitute with pumpkin or sunflower seeds in place of almonds.

PER SERVING (1 tablespoon) Calories: 103; Carbohydrates: 4g; Fat: 9g; Protein: 4g; Fiber: 2g; Sodium: 59mg

STRAWBERRY JAM

Makes 2 cups

PREP TIME: 5 MINUTES / COOK TIME: 20 MINUTES

There are few bigger battles than those over which jam is better—strawberry or grape. I proudly declare myself 100 percent on the strawberry jam side. But no matter what side you fall on, there are few things better than warm bread and fresh jam to eat in the morning. I love how only a few ingredients are needed to make this delicious spread.

2 cups strawberries, fresh or frozen

1 tablespoon chia seeds

1 tablespoon raw sugar

1. In a medium saucepan over medium-high heat, add the strawberries, chia seeds, and sugar. Stir occasionally with a wooden spoon, breaking up the strawberries into little pieces. Once the mixture reaches a boil, reduce the heat to low and let it simmer for 15 to 20 minutes, stirring frequently, until it reaches a jam-like consistency.

2. Remove the pan from the heat and completely cool the jam before storing.

MAKE-AHEAD TIP: Store in an airtight container in the refrigerator for up to 3 months.

PER SERVING (1 tablespoon) Calories: 7; Carbohydrates: 1g; Fat: 0g; Protein: 0g; Fiber: 0g; Sodium: 0mg

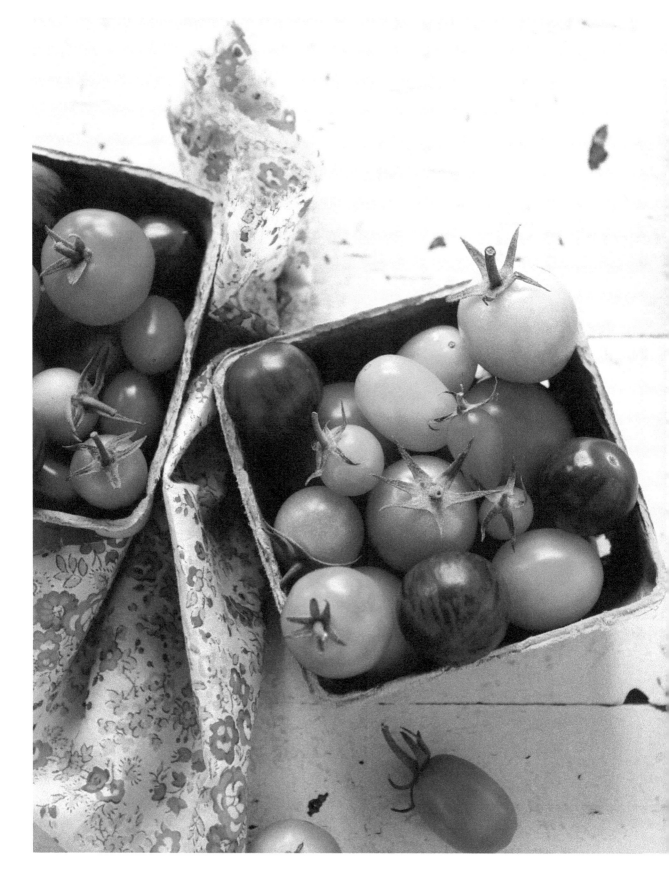

Resources

88 Acres (88Acres.com)
Their Seednola granola, Chocolate & Sea Salt bar, and seed butters are all FODMAP safe and absolutely delicious. The bars are my go-to snacks, and I carry one with me at all times.

Deliberate Fare (DeliberateFare.com)
A wonderful collection of delicious recipes for people following the low-FODMAP diet, as well as people seeking migraine and auto-immune relief.

The Flexible FODMAP Diet Cookbook by Laura Manning, RD, and Karen Frazier (Berkeley, CA: Rockridge Press, 2016)
An excellent recipe book and guide to managing IBS symptoms.

The FODMAP Friendly Food Program (FODMAPfriendly.com)
This is the only organization with a registered trademark certifying FODMAP-safe foods.

Glutino (Glutino.com)
Gluten-free pretzels and other low-FODMAP snacks that taste great.

Healthy Gut, Flat Stomach by Danielle Capalino (Woodstock, VT: Countryman Press, 2017)
A helpful guide with recipes written for the low-FODMAP diet.

Irritable Bowel Syndrome Self Help and Support Group (IBSgroup.org /ibsassociation.org)
A source of information, self-help, and support for all things IBS.

Jovial (JovialFoods.com)
This brand makes some great gluten-free and low-FODMAP pastas and other foods.

A Little Bit Yummy (aLittleBitYummy.com)
This site is full of helpful articles and delicious, dietitian-approved low-FODMAP recipes.

Kate Scarlata (KateScarlata.com)
Kate Scarlata is a registered dietitian who follows a low-FODMAP diet and has popularized the diet in the United States. She provides recipes and other resources for low-FODMAP followers.

Monash University (med.monash.edu/cecs /gastro/fodmap)
This Australian university pioneered the low-FODMAP diet, and they provide wonderful resources regarding all things FODMAP, including frequently updated food guides and research results.

Nutrition for Balance (NutritionForBalance.com)
The website of Gabriela Gardner, a registered and licensed dietitian providing individualized counseling and services.

Measurement Conversions

VOLUME EQUIVALENTS (LIQUID)

US STANDARD	US STANDARD (ounces)	METRIC (approximate)
2 tablespoons	1 fl. oz.	30 mL
¼ cup	2 fl. oz.	60 mL
½ cup	4 fl. oz.	120 mL
1 cup	8 fl. oz.	240 mL
1½ cups	12 fl. oz.	355 mL
2 cups or 1 pint	16 fl. oz.	475 mL
4 cups or 1 quart	32 fl. oz.	1 L
1 gallon	128 fl. oz.	4 L

OVEN TEMPERATURES

FAHRENHEIT (F)	CELSIUS (C) (approximate)
250°F	120°C
300°F	150°C
325°F	165°C
350°F	180°C
375°F	190°C
400°F	200°C
425°F	220°C
450°F	230°C

VOLUME EQUIVALENTS (DRY)

US STANDARD	METRIC (approximate)
⅛ teaspoon	0.5 mL
¼ teaspoon	1 mL
½ teaspoon	2 mL
¾ teaspoon	4 mL
1 teaspoon	5 mL
1 tablespoon	15 mL
¼ cup	59 mL
⅓ cup	79 mL
½ cup	118 mL
⅔ cup	156 mL
¾ cup	177 mL
1 cup	235 mL
2 cups or 1 pint	475 mL
3 cups	700 mL
4 cups or 1 quart	1 L

WEIGHT EQUIVALENTS

US STANDARD	METRIC (approximate)
½ ounce	15 g
1 ounce	30 g
2 ounces	60 g
4 ounces	115 g
8 ounces	225 g
12 ounces	340 g
16 ounces or 1 pound	455 g

The Dirty Dozen and the Clean Fifteen

The Environmental Working Group (EWG) is a nonprofit, nonpartisan organization dedicated to protecting human health and the environment. Its mission is to empower people to live healthier lives in a healthier environment. This organization publishes an annual list of the 12 kinds of produce, in sequence, that have the highest amount of pesticide residue—the Dirty Dozen—as well as a list of the 15 kinds of produce that have the least amount of pesticide residue—the Clean Fifteen.

THE DIRTY DOZEN

The 2016 Dirty Dozen includes the following produce. These are considered among this year's most important produce to buy organically:

1. Strawberries
2. Apples
3. Nectarines
4. Peaches
5. Celery
6. Grapes
7. Cherries
8. Spinach
9. Tomatoes
10. Bell peppers
11. Cherry tomatoes
12. Cucumbers

+ Kale/collard greens*
+ Hot peppers*

*The Dirty Dozen list contains two additional items—kale/collard greens and hot peppers—because they tend to contain trace levels of highly hazardous pesticides.

THE CLEAN FIFTEEN

Items on the Clean Fifteen list are least critical to buy organic. The following are on the 2016 list:

1. Avocado
2. Corn
3. Pineapples
4. Cabbage
5. Sweet peas
6. Onions
7. Asparagus
8. Mangos
9. Papayas
10. Kiwifruit
11. Eggplant
12. Honeydew
13. Grapefruit
14. Cantaloupe
15. Cauliflower

References

American Heart Association. "Fish and Omega-3 Fatty Acids." Accessed May 2017. Web: www.heart.org /HEARTORG/HealthyLiving /HealthyEating/ HealthyDietGoals /Fish-and-Omega-3-Fatty-Acids _UCM_303248_Article.jsp#. WShRvVKZPVo.

Barrett J.S. "Extending Our Knowledge of Fermentable, Short-Chain Cargohydrates for Managing Gastrointestinal Symptoms." *Nutrition in Clinical Practice* 28.3 (2013).

Bohm M., Siwiec R., and Wo J.M. "Diagnosis and Management of Small Intestinal Bacterial Overgrowth." *Nutrition in Clinical Practice* 28.3 (2013).

Catsos, Patsy. "Five Low FODMAP Diet Pitfalls (and What You Can Do to Avoid Them)." International Foundation for Functional Gastrointestinal Disorders. December 24, 2016. Accessed May 2017. Web: www .aboutibs.org/low-fodmap-diet /five-low-fodmap-diet-pitfalls-and -what-you-can-do-to-avoid-them.

Crohn's & Colitis Foundation. "What Are Crohn's & Colitis?" Accessed May 2017. Web: www.crohnscolitisfoundation .org/ what-are-crohns-and-colitis.

Dr. Axe: Food Is Medicine. "Eggplant Nutrition, Benefits & Recipes." Accessed May 2017. Web: www.draxe .com/eggplant-nutrition.

Dukowicz A.C., Lacy B.E., and Levine G.M. "Small Intestinal Bacterial Overgrowth: A Comprehensive Review." *Gastroenterology & Hepatology* 3.2 (2007): 112-22. Web: www.ncbi.nlm.nih .gov/pmc/articles/PMC3099351.

Gearry, Richard B. "Reduction of dietary poorly absorbed short-chain carbohydrates (FODMAPs) improves abdominal symptoms in patients with inflammatory bowel disease—a pilot study." Journal of Crohn's and Colitis (2009).

Gibson P.R., Shepherd S.J. "Evidence-Based Dietary Management of Functional Gastrointestinal Symptoms: The FODMAP Approach." *Journal of Gastroenterology and Hepatology* 25.2 (2010).

IBS Diets: FODMAP Dieting Guide. "FODMAP Food List." Accessed May 2017. Web: www.ibsdiets.org/fodmap -diet/ fodmap-food-list.

International Foundation for Functional Gastrointestinal Disorders. "Celiac Disease." Accessed May 2017. Web: www.iffgd.org/other-disorders/celiac -disease.html.

International Foundation for Functional Gastrointestinal Disorders. "Facts About IBS." Accessed May 2017. Web: www.aboutibs.org/155-what-is-ibs /facts-about-ibs.html.

Mansueto P., Seidita A., D'Alcamo A., and Carroccio A. "Role of FODMAPs in Patients With Irritable Bowel Syndrome." *Nutrition in Clinical Practice* 30.5 (2015).

Mayo Clinic. "Inflammatory Bowel Disease (IBD)." February 18, 2015. Accessed May 2017. Web: www .mayoclinic.org/diseases-conditions /inflammatory-bowel-disease/basics /definition/con-20034908.

Monash University. "Low FODMAP Diet for Irritable Bowel Syndrome." Accessed May 2017. Web: www.med .monash.edu/cecs/gastro/fodmap.

Mullin G.E., Shepherd S.J., Chander Roland B, et al. "Irritable Bowel Syndrome: Contemporary Nutrition Management Strategies." *Journal of Parenteral and Enteral Nutrition* 38.7 (2014).

Shah N., Parian A., Mullin G., and Limketkai B. "Oral Diets and Nutrition Support for Inflammatory Bowel Disease: What Is the Evidence?" *Nutrition in Clinical Practice* 30.4 (2015).

Stepaniak, Jo. "Low FODMAP and Vegan: What to Eat When You Can't Eat Anything. Summertown, TN: Book Publishing, 2016.

Thomas, J. Reggie, Rakesh Nanda, and Lin H. Shu. "A FODMAP Diet Update: Craze or Credible?" *Practical Gastroenterology* 36.12 (2012). Accessed May 2017. Web: www.med .virginia.edu/ginutrition/wp-content /uploads/sites/199/2014/06/Parrish _Dec_12.pdf.

Recipe Index

Index

About the Authors

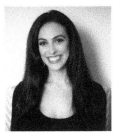

Mollie Tunitsky is a passionate chef, baker, and food blogger who believes that we all have the power to enjoy food and live a healthy, fulfilling life. After many painful years of misdiagnosed stomach issues, discomfort at restaurants, and being told to "avoid this" and "stay away from that," Mollie's journey to health and wellness led her to the low-FODMAP diet. By making smart, simple modifications to her diet, Mollie transformed mealtime from an anxiety-inducing affair to the most enjoyable part of her day. Cooking became fun again as Mollie challenged herself to be creative and resourceful while making new recipes that would not result in digestive issues. Today Mollie lives a less restricted lifestyle and has discovered new FODMAP-safe foods she loves to eat and incorporate into her recipes. Learn how to make FODMAPs work for you and join the community at FitFabFODMAP.com. Mollie lives a fit, fab lifestyle with her husband in Houston, Texas.

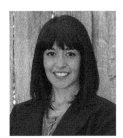

Gabriela Gardner is a Registered Dietitian Nutritionist with certifications in Advanced Practice in Clinical Nutrition and Nutrition Support. Her practice specializes in digestive disorders and she has been published in the journal *Nutrition in Clinical Practice*. She speaks regularly at nutrition and digestive disease conferences, and has been interviewed by Univision, Fox, and Telemundo, as well as on several radio stations. During Gabriela's free time she enjoys practicing yoga and lives a gluten-free lifestyle with her husband in Houston, Texas. For more information about her nutrition practice, visit NutritionForBalance.com.

CPSIA information can be obtained
at www.ICGtesting.com
Printed in the USA
JSHW061918260922
31009JS00004B/9